CUTTINGEDGE

First published in Great Britain in 2004
by Artnik
341b Queenstown Road
London SW8 4LH
UK

© Artnik 2004

ISBN 1 903906 50 4

Design: Mark Lloyd
Edited: Owen O'Rourke
Picture Credits: Rex Features

Printed and bound in Spain by Cayfosa

CUTTING**EDGE**

Laurence Kirwan M.D. F.R.C.S.

ARTNIK

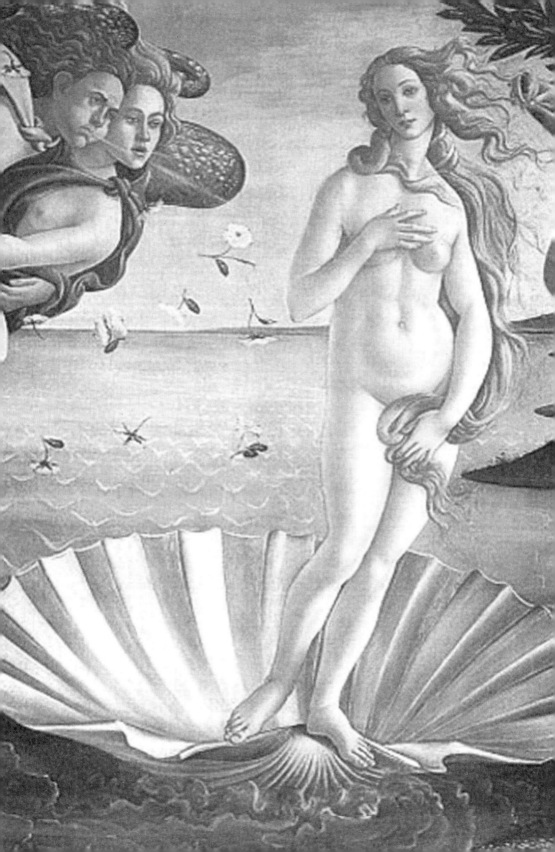

CONTENTS

INTRODUCTION

This book performs a biopsy on contemporary ideals of beauty. It explores the effects of fashion, photography and the media on how we as a society have come to define beauty – more specifically it examines how the effects of plastic surgery, as well as advanced non-surgical procedures, are revolutionising our ideals of the human body.

How does the beauty revolution affect us culturally? How does such artificial self-improvement sit with Darwin? By a form of not-so-natural selection, we are creating an evolutionary imperative whereby beautiful people demand the same in a partner. Women who are independent financially don't pick a man based simply on his ability to provide a home and security. They want a partner that is fun in bed and looks good at the dinner table. Every part of the male and female body has its model of perfection, an aesthetic ideal that we are all either striving to achieve or choosing to ignore. Surgical tweaking may produce results ever closer to these ideals – but this process cannot affect evolution.

The reality is that the 'beautiful' people – driven, ambitious, rich – do not necessarily have more babies. Non-Western cultures, some of which allow multiple wives, are far more reproductive, while placing little or no emphasis on aspiring to our physical ideals. And the great irony of 'evolution' by plastic surgery is this: two people with cute surgically-enhanced noses could marry and have children with big noses. The children of course grow up to look like their parents did before they had surgery, and we see this happen time after time. Nonetheless, many of those who do resort to plastic surgery have a disproportionate influence on society generally – a lot of them literally do set the tone for the rest of us.

In the light of such changes – and it's a very recent development – *Cutting Edge* is my attempt as a practising cosmetic surgeon to describe how this is shaping our aesthetics of the body. I also try to map out how it is influencing our cultural landscape. Although I look in detail at current surgical procedures, I consider the influence of diet and exercise, too. The relatively new fad for health clubs has literally changed the shape of both sexes – we are creating a nation of breastless women – the thin and over-exercised breed. To see the difference, just ogle the screen idols of the fifties: women like Grace Kelly and Sophia Loren, men like Johnny Weismuller as Tarzan. Along the way, the celebrities of today come under my imaginary scalpel – but a simple look at the fashion industry, at magazine covers and shop-window mannequins, is equally revealing. These are the aesthetic standards we live by today.

If you visit the Roman Antiquities Room at the Metropolitan Museum of Art, then walk the short distance to Saks on Fifth Avenue (New York's other 'museum'), you go from where you look at the art to where you can try on the artworks, buy them and take them home. Here you do not simply admire the art – you acquire images that you use as templates to remodel yourself.

Laurence Kirwan
2004

Dedication

To Maurice Kirwan (Morry), my dad 1921-2003, Physician and Surgeon.

He always wanted to see the 21st Century and he did. He used to say that

I wasn't a real doctor because I was a plastic surgeon. Dad was a real doctor.

With love.

And to my wife Chelsea who has endured the aggravation of my spending time in front of

the computer screen instead of time together. If my children read this I hope they enjoy it,

all seven of them, Rony, Dimity, Emma,Francesca, Sebastian, Felicity and Lilibet.

Acknowledgements:

Thanks to my publisher, Valentina, who managed to make this concept a reality in a very short period of time. I will miss our little ménages a trois, just you, me and a digital recorder- and your phone calls to the United States at 8.00 am on Saturday and Sunday mornings. Also my thanks to both Owen O'Rourke who was far too talented for this task and John McVicar who was much too cerebral for my efforts. Without the efforts of both, the book would have been a draft only.

Frederick J. McCoy and Alan Chandler my professors and many others such as Donald Wood-Smith, Marco Gasparotti, Ivo Pitanguy, Yves-Gerard Illouz, Sherrell Aston, Daniel Baker and Joshua Halpern.

Author's note:

Except where specified, the terms 'cosmetic surgery' and 'plastic surgery' are used interchangeably. If they ever had a separate and distinct meaning it has become obscured through usage. Note also that when the book refers to patients, in almost all cases they may be understood to be female. This is because women still constitute 95% of all clients in this industry.

OUT OF **THE CAVE** – HOW IT ALL BEGAN

An introduction: the grooming instinct

In 1967, a zoologist named Desmond Morris published a book called *The Naked Ape*. It was a runaway success, translated into 23 languages, and is still selling. Morris's trick was to write about humans as if they were animals, thereby creating a zoological portrait of our species. The title comes from the fact that of 193 different types of primate on Earth, we are the only one that is relatively hairless. Morris himself was more hairless than most – nearly bald, in fact. To hide the fact, and in the effort actually drawing attention to his own nakedness, he had a giant 'comb-over' *à la* Rudolph Guiliani to cover his shiny pate. Nowadays, given all the money that he earned, Morris would almost certainly have had a hair transplant. Guiliani got an image consultant and wisely opted, with a short back and side, for coming out bald gracefully… for him there will be no going back.

Perhaps a more telling feature of our species is not our comparative hairlessness, but the way we have always adorned, primped and fashioned our bodies. Nowhere is man found actually naked in the sense of being unadorned. Even before clothes were ever made, primitive man put paint on his body, bones in his nose, sand plates in his lips and so on. We are more a fashion-conscious ape than a naked one.

Today adornment in its many facets sends out infinitely more complex social, emotional and cultural signals. Our grooming habits deliver a subtly coded message to the world around us – whether we are conscious of this or not. Men and women display their social status and personal success through a measure of adornment. They strive to project an image that would impress their own peers – as well as attracting a partner.

The way a man dresses sends out signals that pertain to who he is: his age and occupation, how seriously he takes himself, or how he responds to the expectations of others. Typically, women invest in fashionable clothes, make up, hair styling, jewellery and more commonly than men, plastic surgery. In social settings, plastic surgery is an adornment which sets a dividing line between those who have had it and those who haven't. These days the cocktail set can spot someone who didn't get their Botox shot when it was properly due. The cult of youth and beauty has translated into an obsession with every conceivable form of self-enhancement.

Men and women use cosmetic surgery because of the powerful need to conform to expectations. Teenagers sport hipsters and mobile phones. Sloanes drive around with boxes of La Perla lingerie spilling out of the back of their Porsches. No matter what their background, everyone must belong to one or other clearly identifiable set. For some groups, such as Jewish teenagers in North London or New York's Scarsdale a rhinoplasty is just as essential as the mobile phone or the 3 Series BMW convertible.

Moreover, the older and more affluent we grow, the greater the need to compete in our appearance. Extreme youth is unselfconscious; a sense of self-image, and all its problems, arrives as we begin to age. As we become older, we may tend to look more contrived and 'produced' in our pursuit of physical perfection. And yet the best plastic surgery is undetectable, which explains its attraction to many women.

In women, the need to compete is proportionate to how attractive they are (or have been). It may be fuelled by men's propensity to look at, or just notice other women, whether in the pages of a newspaper or in the street. In the 1996 film *The Mirror Has Two Faces*, a plain, overweight woman (Barbra Streisand) resolves to alter her appearance dramatically in the mistaken belief that her husband does not find her sexually attractive. Once she achieves the desired transformation, she is lectured by a friend: 'From now on, you will watch everything you eat. You will go on shopping expeditions and monitor fashion magazines. Most importantly, every time you walk into a room, you will scour it for faces that might possibly be more attractive than yours.' The modern woman understands this instinctively.

Both men and women of a certain age may fall into the trap of clinging on to their vanishing youth, rather than cultivating individuality and sophistication. Uniqueness is the single most powerful currency in the looks department, yet this is frequently undervalued. Striving for flawlessness and uniformity of image will continue to drive cosmetic surgery, and further widen the divide between the beautiful people and those 'afflicted' by old age, imperfection – and a lack of funds to do anything about it.

This book does not say that ageing is unacceptable: it is something we cannot prevent so to some extent we must embrace it. Tommy Lee Jones and Barbara Hepburn, amongst many others, have proudly weathered the storms of age without a visit to the plastic surgeon. But this book is for those who *are* interested in cosmetic surgery – whether you are for or against makes no difference. Those against are often the most interested.

It is not unusual for me to be accosted at some cocktail party by a woman – and it *is* usually a woman – and accused of being a propagator of the addiction called plastic surgery. She will go into great detail on why she considers it so offensive.

Just as I would never initiate such a discussion, nor would I object to it. For those of us in the plastic surgery field, it does at least show that our patients are not the only ones affected by and fascinated with what we do.

The origins of cosmetic surgery

Cosmetic surgery sprang from multiple branches of medicine. The most recent origins of plastic surgery date from the First World War when American and European surgeons worked in military hospitals on the injured soldiers, rebuilding their faces. However, the very first rhinoplasty, or 'nose job', was performed by Dr. Jacques Joseph in Germany in 1898. Dr. Gustav Aufricht, an Austrian surgeon (but also, like Joseph, a Romanian Jew) is then credited with bringing the procedure to the United States in the 1930s.

The American Board of Plastic Surgery, Inc. was established in June 1937 by representatives of various groups involved with this type of surgery, and then received recognition as a subsidiary of the American Board of Surgery in May 1938. The ABPS was given the status of a major speciality board in May 1941 by action of the Advisory Board for Medical Specialities (ABMS), which designates certain fields as being suitable for representation by speciality boards. There is only one Board of Plastic Surgery recognised by the ABMS.

Plastic surgery was further advanced during the Second World War, particularly in England where many Spitfire pilots were badly burnt in their cockpits. This was mainly a result of their orders to land a burning plane since planes were in such short supply rather than use a parachute and ditch it. One of the most notable surgeons at the time was Sir Harold Gillies. Many other surgeons worked during this period and took their experience home to Europe and the United States. However, many of the procedures we are so conversant with today, such as liposuction and breast enlargement, simply did not exist then. Others were still in their early stages, such as tummy-tucks and facelifts.

Yet even with these early advances in the field of cosmetic surgery there was one astonishing gap – the absence of a good medical text on the subject. This was remedied in 1976 when Tom Rees wrote *Aesthetic Plastic Surgery*, which remains a good reference work, still consulted by professionals in the field.

This book was to become an early milestone in cosmetic surgery. Hard as it is for us to believe, cosmetic surgery was until then considered far too unimportant to merit specialised study, and not even recognised as a speciality in the field of surgery. People who practiced it were on the fringes of the larger field of plastic surgery. Now the opposite is true: the purely reconstructive plastic surgeon is being relegated to second place behind the cosmetic practitioner.

Within another 20 years or less, plastic surgery as a reconstructive art will be a forgotten specialist field. This trend has been dictated by US insurance companies, who have created a climate where plastic surgeons are not adequately reimbursed for what are often very lengthy, complex and difficult operations. As a result, thousands of doctors have moved on to non-insurance based practices – essentially cash practices. This, in turn, has driven plastic surgeons out of reconstructive surgery, which is now almost solely performed in University settings in the US and by the NHS in this country.

Thus, in the future, plastic surgery will be synonymous with cosmetic surgery – but in terms of the gold standard, because of the depth and scope of his training, the plastic surgeon is and will remain the best qualified person to operate. The process of qualification is long and arduous and the job itself very demanding. In the United States, most plastic surgeons are required to complete not only their basic medical training but also a full surgical training program in General Surgery Orthopaedics or Ear, Nose and Throat Surgery before completing a full training program in Plastic Surgery. Many surgeons go on to do a further year in a specialised area of plastic surgery such as Hand Surgery or cosmetic surgery.

At the moment the speciality is still practised mainly by men whose patients are still mainly women. This is just a plain statement of fact, which has no sexist undertones.

Cosmetic surgery has recently enjoyed a dramatic expansion for a number of reasons, none of which are connected to advances in medicine. While it is true that medicine in general has made dramatic progress in the last century (we have sterility of the surgical environment, anaesthesia, blood transfusions, antibiotics and safer surgery), the reasons for plastic surgery's unprecedented popularity are entirely due to changes in society itself.

Consider this: a baby boomer turns 50 years of age every 8 seconds.

We in the West have been living through an era of unprecedented affluence. Until the terrorist threats of the last few years, it has also been one without fear. Whereas previous generations lived under the shadow of war or the looming threat of a nuclear holocaust, our concerns now tend to be localised. We worry far more about our social status or what are the prospects in our career or how much money we earn than we do about, for example, global warming. We have, so to speak, become free to explore our inner space and our private selves. We are not merely a part of the 'me generation' – we are in the 'me zone'.

The free world is more interested in making dollars than acquiring empires. There is a surge of capitalist societies and every capitalist society is driven by free-spending consumers. There are only so many things one can buy – a house, a car, clothes – all status symbols and adornments. But no amount of dripping diamonds or Versace gear will hide the saggy neck or bags under the eyes: after a while it becomes obvious when mutton is being dressed as lamb. Plastic surgery is a logical continuation of the consumerist drive, the next big must-have for the ageing material girl.

This to some degree explains the huge increase in cosmetic surgery and why it is definitely here to stay. The underlying peer pressure comes from the media: magazines, newspapers and, ever more so, television and film.

Ethical considerations

People who practice medicine should, of course, be motivated more by altruistic reasons than monetary ones. Certainly, this is the case in the UK where NHS doctors' salaries are no more than adequate. In the States, however, as medicine is practised much more in the private sector and most doctors make a much better living, the fulcrum is more towards the financial. In respect of plastic surgery, most people assume its practitioners are driven solely by money.

Yet, plastic surgery is equally as laudable as mainstream medicine. We don't cure disease or heal injury but, in the round, we improve the quality of people's lives equally as much. Whether you are fixing a cleft palate, reconstructing a breast or doing a facelift, the emphasis is on improving the way people feel about themselves and can relate towards others. The difference, of course, is that while the NHS funds reconstructive surgery, cosmetic surgery is, for the time being, privately funded. Incidentally, many a plastic surgeon has operated for charity – but a facelift is never seen in itself as a charitable contribution. Nonetheless, it can do as much good to the patient as removing an unsightly facial birthmark or burn.

Motivations for plastic surgery:

Sexual attraction

A basic human motivation is to look better in order to appeal to the opposite sex – this is what drives fashion, make-up and plastic surgery. Having said that, the gay community are big consumers of plastic surgery, and are also makers and shakers of fashion and style – so let's just say it's the basic motive to appeal to the person we find sexually attractive, according to whatever our preferences may be.

Much has been written on the subject of why women resort to plastic surgery. The conventional wisdom is that they do so in order to please their partners and acquire confidence. Women who have lived with the same man for a long time often complain their partner becomes immune to their looks – even if they are very attractive. There is certainly a great deal of truth in that. But no woman rushes off to the plastic surgeon because her husband has said something like, 'Darling, I think you look awful, I think you should have something done.' She leaves him first, then *after* the divorce settlement she goes to see a plastic surgeon.

Certainly, men love their partners for many reasons other than the fact that they may be a stunning beauty. A man's ego may receive a considerable boost when he walks into a room with a beautiful woman on his arm, but ultimately – and contrary to what many women seem to believe – that is not what their man wants most from them. It is their cuddles, the kisses, the affection, even their conversation. Women may complain that their husbands are the last ones to notice any change in their appearance. This is true, but most of us do not scrutinise other people's faces in any great detail – a fact frequently ignored by men as well as women. We spend a great deal of time examining our own faces and bodies believing that the world at large is aware of every little spot or imperfection. In fact, the opposite is true. Men can shave off their moustaches and women fail to notice; the same is even truer of men when women dye their hair.

The reasons for considering plastic surgery are myriad. Women mostly do it for themselves – and occasionally to make their husbands happy, on the understanding that their husbands would never make such a request themselves. But they might also do it because they are in an unhappy marriage. The scenario of a husband who is never there, leaving his wife to shop and spend money by way of recreation, is all too frequent. Once their wives have bought all the furs, clothes and jewellery they care to, they start bleeding money on the operating table.

Ageing

There are people who get divorced and suddenly, after 30 years of marriage, are no longer 'invisible' – they see themselves in the mirror with new eyes and begin to feel as if their happiness is controlled by their external image. None of us want to have a lifestyle that is limited by our age. None of us want to be defined by our age. Many of my older patients refuse to tell people their real age, for fear of being subtly shunted out of their social circle.

Then, there are the career women who have to work hard not to be bypassed because of the unprecedented climate of ageism we are seeing today. Most of us celebrate youth culture but the other side of the coin is ageism.

Self-image

Plastic surgery changes lives. I like to cite the example of a patient of mine – an English nanny – who went from having a biker boyfriend to a banker boyfriend as a result of simple nose surgery. The result changed not only her appearance, but her entire life, in that it gave her the confidence to interact with a different social group. The effect of the surgery was more than external – it changed the way she felt about herself.

It does not necessarily follow that people who have plastic surgery to improve their looks are guaranteed more interesting and successful lives. There are people whose lives were boring and tedious before and will be boring and tedious after any amount of surgical enhancement. But there are people whose lives will change significantly as a result of surgery, and much of it has to do with attitude – both their own and that of others.

On the other hand, plastic surgery is often a simple question of a person's self-mage not measuring up to the challenges of new circumstances. People might want to look good at a high school re-union, or as the mother of the bride, or even the mother, who was late having a child, on the first day of school. It can come down to quite mundane considerations…or so it may seem to others. There are the middle-aged women who have lost breast volume after childbirth or whose tummies protrude after pregnancy; and there are women who would like to get back into a nice dress or a bikini and wear fashionable clothes instead of big jumpers.

Conformity

The person seeking cosmetic surgery is not interested in its relationship to ethics – rather, they are interested in its relationship to beauty, as defined by those people who grace the covers of magazines.

I think the National Portrait Gallery should, in the next century, be full of magazine covers – and images of the cover girls who sell the magazines. What sells is an image of a person who typifies something others aspire to be. In their own time, portraits of the Duke of Wellington, Admiral Nelson and Bonaparte were popular for these reasons. Nowadays women open magazines because they covet the model's looks, both her body and her clothes. They don't care what, if anything, is in her head. Naomi Campbell may be viewed by many as a drug-addicted nincompoop but she sells magazines because she looks sensational.

As trends change, so do the faces on the covers of magazines – and the ones hanging on people's walls. It is interesting that the Royal Academy recently ran an exhibition of Pre-Raphaelite Art. The revival of the figurative painting's last great stand, boasting exquisitely beautiful women with large lips and eyes, shows how our interest in Art History reflects our tastes in beauty today.

Peer Pressure

I have patients who feel comfortable with the way they look yet resolve to have a facelift, for example, because their peers look substantially younger as a result of cosmetic surgery.

We can draw an analogy here between going for plastic surgery and driving a Ferrari. Why do we buy Ferraris? To keep up with the Joneses – perhaps to overtake the Joneses. They're fun to drive but mostly we want the buzz from everyone turning to look at us. There's not much room in the back, it's not particularly comfortable – you can't really even go faster than anyone else, not when driving around a city like London... yet we feel better because everyone around us is saying in so many ways that we *must* feel better. In fact, contrary to the received intellectual wisdom, a lot of the things we are told will make us feel better, actually do so. People around us define our situation much more definitively than we do – being admired and envied makes one feel worthy of being admired and envied. This is the way that humans tick, and it's so strong that when someone has something that others admire and envy, by and large, they flaunt it.

Say you have a Ferrari: to confirm that this pain-of-a-city car is worthwhile, you drive up and down the Santa Monica Boulevard, basking in all the admiration and envy. This became so popular – there are more Ferraris in Beverley Hills than Turin or, for that matter, Medellin – that you could walk faster than the cars were moving. The tailbacks became so bad that the police blocked off the Boulevard at night to stop the Ferrari-drivers picking up their ego-fix. In the pre-automobile age, the Kensington Gore was its own Santa Monica Boulevard and, in some Romantic Latin towns, the populace still promenades in the evening to admire and pay homage to the beauties, both cars *and* women.

There is peer pressure and, then, there is business pressure – people don't want to be laid off for the way they look. It is no longer a question of *Keep young and beautiful if you want to be loved*, more like, Keep young and beautiful, if you want to be *employed*.

The film industry is the obvious example of this, and not just the stars: most executive vice-presidents are in their early 30s controlling multi-million dollar budgets. The record industry is the same, as is the banking industry...in both sectors it is rare to find managing directors in their late forties. By then, they are usually either retired or fired. This, sadly is the reality we have to live with, and it applies to everyone. Look at the people we elect into the top jobs: George W. Bush and William Jefferson Clinton are both still in their fifties, and Tony Blair is only fifty-one. In contrast, Churchill was sixty-five when he first became Prime Minister.

In recent years, there has been a definitive trend to start using cosmetic surgery in order to correct or alter one's appearance before we even start to sag or age. Boys and girls typically start to want rhinoplasty in their teens. In fact only 50% of my practice is devoted to rejuvenation: the rest are patients who want to alter or enhance their appearance. The line between rejuvenating and corrective surgery is becoming more and more blurred today, because many procedures once used to make people look younger are also procedures used for changing the way we look, period.

BEAUTY THROUGH
THE AGES

Fantasy, myth, and how to avoid looking like your mother

I f beauty is in the eye of the beholder, is the beholder a male or female? Until very recently, the male beholder certainly defined our social version of beauty. But how has this perception arisen?

A woman is an object of attention: men look at women and women are aware of it. When a woman walks into a room, she is observed and the observers are men. Consider how the female form has been the subject of so much figurative art. Women, often nude women, have been painted for men to admire. Similarly most pornography caters for male tastes because – to give it a positive spin – the female face and body have always been seen as something to admire. That is an historical truth, and that is why so much art is representational of women. The men pay for it and the women pose: Hugh Hefner and Larry Flint understood this instinctively, and didn't require a lengthy rationale.

The reasons men chase good-looking women are rooted deep in our biology. We know attractiveness is a desirable asset, but what is it that defines the physically attractive?

Does it have to be supermodel good looks or is it just being well presented? It's a mixture of both, of course. Even supermodels have their physical imperfections and you can see, in how they dress, that most of them are observing the 'What not to wear' rules so as to maximise the good parts and minimise the bad.

When men are attracted to women, it is not necessarily for the purpose of reproducing with them, which limits the credibility of the biological conditioning argument. Of course, men are more attracted to sex for its own pleasurable sake than women since, amongst other things, they don't have the babies. And they are aroused by the obvious parts of the female body that signal sexual pleasure: their lips, their breasts, their buttocks. This was all determined by nature a long time before you and I arrived on the scene but even allowing for the fact that beauty is not all that matters it does carry some biological weight.

This book sets out to examine the importance of physical beauty because, even though beauty isn't everything, it is one of the strongest fixations of the human species.

Perceptions are everything

Changing your appearance can dramatically change your life.

Even though many of us are loath to acknowledge it, the way we look affects the way we feel. Some people seem reluctant to accept the self-evident fact that we all engage in a certain amount of grooming for the specific purpose of looking better – women put on make-up, men put on a nice suit or its informal equivalent, women have their hair done, men shave, and so on.

Personally, I find that looking better makes me feel better. If I look like a slob, I feel like a slob. This can be extended all the way to superstardom and supermodels, and it is the driving force behind fashion, make-up and ultimately cosmetic plastic surgery. Consider all forms of basic personal grooming: a decent haircut, perhaps. Look at our hygienic rituals, using razors or make-up, perfumes and creams. Then, there is how we dress in the mornings. The next step on this continuum of looking better is actually changing the physical characteristics of one's body through injections and surgery. Such a step is only different in degree not kind.

Naturally, a person with a perfect body would have no need for that final stage, but they will probably endorse every other stage along the way. Perfect bodies are rare and people who have the confidence to believe in their own physical perfection even more so.

If you want to change your appearance in some perceptible way, you might put on a different lipstick; if a person doesn't have that perfect body, they might go to the next level of plastic surgery. Even those who we'd call perfect have the same insecurities and the same desire to tweak their genetic inheritance.

That is the level at which plastic surgery will continue. It has never been a very accessible option, cost being just one of the impediments to making that step. Surgery has never been trouble-free or pain-free, nor is it even today – but the chances of surgery being made simpler and safer are better today than ever before, and the results are more consistent. What is driving more and more people to the plastic surgeon, beyond the media barrage, is that we can now provide cosmetic surgery at a reasonable cost and reasonable risk level. A look in our magazines, papers and TV listings shows the intense public interest in cosmetic surgery.

The way we look is so important in how others perceive us. Perfectly self-evident as this may sound, it is amazing how many exist in denial – or are not even aware if it.

Deconstructing the perfect body
Throughout history, people have always striven towards a

particular beauty ideal. Today, this ideal is defined by a cabal of the media and fashion industries. To see this ideal personified, all we need do is trawl the high street fashion outlets and look at the mannequins shaped precisely to reflect that beauty ideal. Look at them without their clothes on, 'in the nude' as it were. Sir Kenneth Clark once noted that without our clothes on we are just naked but with posture and attitude nudity becomes an art form.

A passing foray into a regular teenage outlet like FCUK (let alone an up-market one such as Gucci, Prada, Harvey Nicks or Harrods) would suggest clothes are produced for a mannequin's body shape. Sometimes the mannequins are fashioned after famous models, just as Bernini would choose a noted beauty as a model for his sculpture. Fashion models and mannequins are selected to project the beauty ideal of the day. They have similar proportions and model the same clothes. The models of every decade belong to it, and don't seem to weather well in terms of *our* conception of beauty, any better than does a Gainsborough painting.

If fashion didn't reinvent itself, it wouldn't be fashion.
When we try to deconstruct the beauty ideal, we should take a closer look at these fashion shop mannequins and their general proportions: what size breasts and hips they have; how the ankles are turned, the shape of the buttocks. Forgetting the face for now – that's a world in itself – consider other characteristics such as the neck – even the neck!...

Look at the length and the shape of the neck, the nape of the neck: what makes it sexy? We could look at the bottom of the neck where it meets the chest: the 'suprasternal notch', as Ralph Fiennes described it to Kristin Scott-Thomas in *The English Patient*. The attention he pays to this supra-sternal notch is a good example of how *every* part of our physique has an aesthetic ideal that is anchored to its sexual appeal.

We should look at the shoulders and at the upper arms – an area that is very important for women from an aesthetic point of view. The posture of the neck and back also reflects on the way these parts look. A rounded back can spoil an otherwise attractive neck or shoulders.

Most women's forearms and hands are delicate, but their upper arms tend to have a lot of problems – they are often too heavy or even fat in younger women, whereas older women tend to have too much extra skin (that, or they are not developed enough muscularly). Both men and women need to develop muscle in the arms to achieve definition, because that looks sexier. Resistance training or muscle strengthening exercises help women create lean, toned bodies while reducing the flab. The same applies to shoulders, again a muscle definition issue and not a cosmetic surgery one.

Breasts have always been an important erotic symbol and a source of sexual fascination. Consider Greek sculpture such as the Medici

Venus from the 3rd century B.C. (Galleria degli Uffizi, Florence) and Renaissance Art such as Raphael's Three Graces c.1505-06 (Musee Conde, Chantilly). For me one of the most provocative portraits is that of Gabrielle d'Estrees and one of her sisters who is gently and suggestively pinching her right nipple. The allure of breasts is ancient and elusive. Desmond Morris, in The Naked Ape, goes so far as to suggest that they evolved to mimic buttocks, so that intercourse could be conducted face-to-face and not the way the animals did it. Doggy-style was not conducive to the kind of intimacy necessary to bond the couple for the arduous pregnancy and the long period required to bring up a child. The missionary position has its own biological imperative rather than any divine-sanctioned one.

Breasts should be a certain proportionate size; they should be perky and shouldn't sag. I would draw two tongue-in-cheek limits: they should not project forward beyond the point of the chin, and when jogging they should not bounce up and down more than six inches with a normal sport bra! Breasts can of course be made bigger or smaller – or even completely removed. Consider the Amazons, who would remove their right breast to facilitate aiming a bow – or the enforced mastectomy of St Agatha, martyred by Roman soldiers who severed her breasts and then presented them on a platter (perhaps in a crude attempt at breast implants). But these were not aesthetic issues (for my part, I would have redesigned the bow).

The tummy should be flat, but that slight rotundity below the umbilicus is sexy – too flat is too masculine, although there is a tendency now to have a totally flat tummy. One should see a thin line down the middle of the abdomen, but not a six-pack, which again is too masculine – it suggests no fat whatsoever on the abdomen. You want to see a masking of the muscle, yet a little definition coming through.

The bones of the hips should show only at the front. The buttocks should be tight: they shouldn't sag, they should be smooth and there shouldn't be any cellulite. They should also be round not flat. Buttocks have several planes to them: they are flat at the sides, they curve around at the back, and then they curve into the small of the back above. There is a slight indentation at the side of the buttock and then the curve of the buttock underneath should be subtle. There should be a line between the buttock and the thigh, but there is a limit to how marked it should be – if it were too pronounced, it would suggest a degree of sagging. Buttocks should have bounce and they should be round from top to bottom on profile. A fuller *butt* is definitely more fashionable but as with breasts they should not jiggle up and down when walking – and they should not be wider than the thighs.

The thigh should be tight in all directions; it should be curved on the back, flat on the outer and inner sides, and it should have a slight curve on the front. The calves should be narrow at the bottom, thicker but not too thick at the top, and one should be able to see muscle. But remember that too much visible muscle begins to look ugly. This is a trap that a lot of women (particularly those who bodybuild) fall into, because they workout until they have no body fat. Definition is good, but muscle should be draped as if under a thin blanket. Ideally, you don't want to see ribs or hip-bones in a woman – you want to see some smoothness.

The 'mannequin' I have described above is constructed by piecing together all the individual aspects of the physical ideal, as dictated by contemporary standards. Photographers are aware of this concept and have models for different parts of the body, with no one model exemplifying the ideal for all areas. If you want to shoot a picture evoking James Bond holding a gun between a woman's legs, you don't choose a face or a neck model. If you're running an ad about hand-cream, then you commission a hand model. There is always an individual who can best embody a particular part.

Beauty in Art

Long before photography, artists sought to define and immortalise beauty in their work, with painting or sculpture. Artists did not have to invest women with sexuality. Rather, artists who loved women portrayed beautiful women as sexual objects. I want to name some personal favourites.

Boticelli's Primavera 1477-1478 (Galleria degli Uffizi, Florence) and Birth of Venus 1485 (Galleria degli Uffizi, Florence) display a great painter who loved the female shape; a smirking courtesan in the former is still alluring and flirtatious today. Piero di Cosimo portrays a particularly striking Simonetta Vespucci (Musee Conde, Chantilly), a noted Florentine beauty with a perfect profile and long neck.

Michelangelo and Donatello were clearly lovers of men. The sculpture of St George is very effeminate; Michelangelo's breasts resemble walnuts. Such artists mostly glorified the beauty of the male, as personified in the sculpture of David.

In the 19th Century, the invention of photography gave us a new medium for shaping our ideal – one which would outstrip the popularity of figurative art in its ability to celebrate the human shape. Today mass media provides vehicles for these same images, digital and celluloid: our perfect images of beauty are delivered to us daily in magazines and newspapers.

Photography was limited in that it could portray no more than what it saw: it could not alter an image in the way an artist could. Early models and screen goddesses could not be made to look any better than their make-up allowed – and for me the Marilyn Monroe look is dated (Marilyn did have a nose job, but the fullness of her upper body – especially her arms – is unfashionable today). This was in the days before Linda Hamilton of *Terminator* fame (1984) wore her sexy 'wife beater' shirt to show off her toned muscled arms.

What revolutionised human imagery was the development of plastic surgery in second half of the 20th century: an event that was to change, quite literally, the face of beauty. If photography helped shape our image of desirability, then with plastic surgery we actually got under its skin.

An analogy would be that when the Eiffel Tower was built, we were able to get a view of our surroundings that is now commonplace from any airplane. Equally when we first saw the world from space we became a small blue planet in the middle of a vast emptiness and a new paradigm was born.

Photography in the 19th Century and then plastic surgery in the 20th Century were equivalent to the Eiffel Tower and the view from the first manned space-craft respectively.

Even though the beauty ideal has altered through the ages, reflecting an artist's subjective taste early on, and the trends of mass media later, what we humans perceive instinctively as attractive owes more to ideal proportion and bone-structure than it does to the ever-changing diktats of fashion. To illustrate this, I make some historical comparisons of five beautiful women of centuries past to those of five women whose faces are in 2004 their fortune.

Ten Faces

To begin with I visited the Greek Room at The Metropolitan Museum of Art on Fifth Avenue, in the heart of New York City. Of course, there are other examples – perhaps the Venus de Milo in the Paris Louvre.

One particular work of art from the 6th century BC, entitled Sabina, represents an aesthetic highpoint in early western civilisation. It is an expression of beauty unencumbered by the religious beliefs that coloured art under the Roman Catholic church. The consummate skill of the artist is clear. There are no rigid lines, only flowing curves, and his mastery of the medium would be unrivalled until Bernini sculpted St Theresa in 1644.

And yet the image is also somewhat static and heavy. There is great beauty in the piece, and when it was first created it would have been painted like an Egyptian mummy, adorned with rich clothing like a FCUK mannequin – but the features remind us of a god-like, rather than a sexual presence. Remember, though, that for the Greeks beauty symbolised goodness.

So on to two great images of beauty: Boticelli's 'Birth of Venus' 1485 (painted for the private residence of the Villa Lorenzi di Pierfrancesco – now in the Uffizi in Florence) and Raphael's 'The Nymph Galatea' 1514 (also in a private residence, the Villa Farnesina in Rome). These figures have heavy limbs and torsos, yet we can see in Venus a similarity to Cindy Crawford and the beginning of an understanding of what constitutes 'timeless' beauty.

I went to the Metropolitan Museum of Art intending to illustrate a point about the fallacy of Greek Art and its expression of beauty. The classical beauty belongs in the time of Greeks: our modern ideal of beauty is better expressed in the interpretations of the Renaissance. Raphael's Galatea and Boticelli's Venus were the supermodels of the 15th and 16th centuries – the art gallery is now their catwalk. Yet in a time before photography we could not have appreciated them without standing in front of the fresco itself (the opposite is now true: it is strange how we think we know so much art through photographs and reproduction, and not in the flesh as it was intended).

The modern-day Galatea and Venus are thinner and their cheeks are more sculpted. But by the 17th Century, we see Bernini creating women such as Daphne with figures that approach starvation, and adolescent features reminiscent of Kate Moss. However, modern art no longer tries to recreate the beauty we see in reality, instead it symbolically explores the mind's eye.

I am standing outside the shop window of Max Mara in the Via Condotti in Rome, no more than a quarter of a mile from Bernini's Fountain in the Piazza Novona. Behind me is the mannequin of a supermodel. How does she differ from Sabina?

Here in the mannequin is the modern-day Praxiteles at work

(Praxiteles was the sculptor of the Goddess of Love in the 4th Century B.C., at the time of the construction of the Acropolis). Like the commercial tailor's dummy, Sabina and the Greek goddesses were painted and clothed to be admired.

This mannequin has no artistic merit. It is a robotic figure, mass-produced with no nipples and no genitals. Nor is there any attempt to convey emotion such as in a work by Bernini. Like a Barbie doll, she is angular and distinguished as a female only by her secondary sexual characteristics. But she is worth studying nonetheless, for this is the image of beauty that should be sitting in the Metropolitan Museum of Art another 2000 years from now. They should mount it next to the bust of Sabina in the Greco-Roman gallery.

Beauty and Race

Humans breed like animals, and we pair off and mate in the same way that we match the stallion to the mare. It's a question of breeding in certain types. We may observe this process on the grandest scale in royalty: the pairing of Prince Charles and Princess Diana, for example. There has admittedly been a recent trend in royalty marrying commoners, something the rest of us do rather less self-consciously.

Most of us are pretty predictable in that we tend to choose people of similar ethnic and social background. Exceptions happen every day, but as a general trend we choose people from the same race and

Images

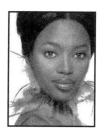
Naomi Campbell born London, 1970 photograph, 1994

Oni from Ife, Nigeria, 12th- 14th century, Museum of Mankind, London
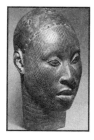

Kate Moss born London 1974 photograph 1992
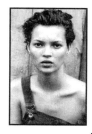

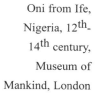
Daphne born 1602 by Gian Lorenzo Bernini for Cardinal Scipione Bhorghese, 1625

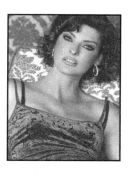
Linda Evangelista born Ontario, 1965, photograph 1997

Constanza Bonarelli born Rome, 1610, by Gian Bernini, 1598 –1680, for himself 1635
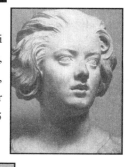

Cindy Crawford born de Kalb, Illinoi,s 1966 photograph 1990
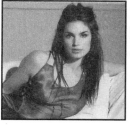

Galatea born 1490 Rome by Raphael Sanzio (1483 – 1520) for the Villa Farnesina Rome 1514

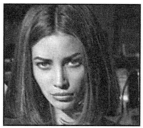
Christie Turlington born Oakland California, photograph 1988

Venus Florence (Italy) by Sandro Boticelli (1446 – 1510) for Lorenzo di Pierfrancesco de' Medici 1485.
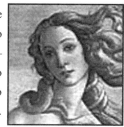

with the same upbringing. This means that we are usually looking at people in our own image in terms of how we perceive beauty.

The classic ignorant comment is that all blacks look the same to whites and vice versa...the same goes for the Asians. Evidently, we recognise features within our own race better than we recognise them in others. But does Will Smith really look like Morgan Freeman, or Jackie Chan like Ken Watanabe? A plastic surgeon has a different approach, because we scrutinise and appreciate different races to a greater extent.

There is beauty in every culture, and every culture celebrates its own. Whether in Japan or Africa, Saudi Arabia or India, there are the famous beauties of their own countries. Anyone looking upon that essential beauty anywhere in the world can see that the women and men who fall into that category are by any standard good-looking. To my eye there are perhaps more beautiful women in some countries than others. From Europe, the northern Italians, the Croatians, the Swiss, French and Scandinavians all spring to mind... but these are personal tastes, and I wouldn't like to offend any nation by their exclusion!

Mixed-race, too, produces combinations that are exciting and attractive. Eurasian women are some of the most beautiful in the world: tall with an olive complexion, an Asian tilt to their eyes and a lack of body hair. This can save on LASER treatment...

CELEBRITY

Or why we all want to have the same nose

There is no excellent beauty that hath not some strangeness in the
proportion — **Francis Bacon, Essays: Of Beauty**

N obody is perfectly beautiful, although certain women are celebrated as being so. People seldom realise that, to begin with, every face is asymmetrical. And beauty is actually perceived in imperfections rather than in perfection. Perfection is cartoonish, like the face of the mannequin – it has a superficial attraction, a degree of aesthetic pleasantness, but it has no human depth. What makes a face interesting is its humanity, its imperfections. The face is the message centre where we project who we are and what we feel. Life, of course – gradually and subtly – puts its imprint on whatever features nature gave us, and some of these imprints the patient will ask the cosmetic surgeon to remove. But I never seek to eradicate all imperfection – faces must always be asymmetrical in order to stay human.

This is why the over-operated face becomes offensive, even repellent to the eye. It can no longer broadcast all those subtle, subliminal messages that are as much a part of communication as actual speech. It feels like you are dealing with an alien or a robot, or being spoken to by a newscaster. The face, then, presents the biggest challenge to the cosmetic surgeon. When I work on the face, I see myself as a cosmetic surgeon AND an artist.

People of both sexes and all ages resort to cosmetic surgery in order to enhance their looks. There is a pre-conceived idea that cosmetic surgery mostly caters for women desperate to retain their youthful looks. This was once the case but it is no longer so. Now there exists far more of a mixed bag of consumers: young men and women who are dissatisfied with the way they have always looked rather than the way they have aged, perhaps. Clearly there are still women who want to turn back the clock but now many men, too, want to reverse the signs of ageing. A shot of Botox is nothing to be ashamed of!

The defiance of ageing

Ageing itself is such a relative term. We can age our body by wild swings in weight and lifestyle as well as excessive sunbathing, smoking, drinking, or even exercise and dieting. In general, exercise and diet will help keep us in shape and defy ageing to some extent. Cosmetic surgery can address issues that exercise and diet alone cannot remedy.

As we get older we usually lose some of the subcutaneous fat on our face and look more skeletal. While it is trendy to look skeletal, this is not necessarily a good thing – the image of youth is to have a nice smooth look with a fuller face. This is derived from the layer of fat beneath the skin, which covers the underlying muscle. As one gets older, this layer is difficult to recreate – excessive weight loss merely compounds the difficulty. Cosmetic surgery cannot do everything... but we are getting there.

There is a section of society that seeks to retain and perfect their youthful looks. Their obsessive drive towards perfection has created something approaching a new breed of people: the super-enhanced who, while growing older, appear not to age. A necessary condition of joining this breed is relatively unlimited funds, and the desire to join – a kind of '*celebrité oblige*' – but what truly marks out the super-enhanced from the rest of us is the quality of eternal youth. Of course, when this is mentioned, the critics begin reaching for their Dorian Gray parallels.

Unlike Dorian Gray, who aged completely when he saw his portrait, there need not be some sudden cataclysmic ageing event when you come due for your next facelift – providing you maintain the look regularly. The startling thing is that women in their sixties, ten years on from their first facelift in their fifties, still look ten years younger than their peers. Until now the give-away has been the hands and décolleté which reveal the true age of the canvas. Yet even these can be corrected. Remember: a continuing relationship with your plastic surgeon is not some Faustian pact with the devil. Agelessness is not bought by selling your soul but by paying your surgeon's fees – although the ancient family heirlooms might have to be sold to achieve it.

In my experience, most who pay the cosmetic surgery piper feel good for what they buy. There are the odd exceptions, of course, because not all surgeons do a good job – or, more commonly, the patient has unrealistic expectations; but, given the effect of our appearance on how others respond to us, it is hardly surprising that people who look better, feel better.

Why celebrities look good

This may surprise a few people – but the single greatest quality that separates us from the vast majority of people in the public eye (especially those whose jobs depend on their looks) is that they've had a LOT of surgery, and that they have it done *all the time*. It is not unusual for celebrities, if that is what we must call them, to have treatments every 6 months to a year – facelifts, nose jobs, eyes tightened, cheek implants, Botox and so on. They have to, otherwise they would simply not look anywhere near as beautiful or young as they do.

The question of whether people in the public eye have had cosmetic surgery is thus obsolete. It is rather a question of *when* and *what* rather than if: and frankly the few that haven't would be well advised to. A radical change every ten years is much more likely to attract the revealing shots of the paparazzi than a regular maintenance programme that leaves you always looking good and at your best. This involves frequent surgery but, when you're under constant scrutiny, you won't want to age into something dreadful and then suddenly come back looking dramatically different. This is what turns you into a humiliating spread in the *News of the World*.

Farah Fawcett is a good recent example of this – the change in her face was so dramatic that it was obvious to everybody she'd had a facelift. What compounded it was that the after the operation, the nasal tip was a ball and the nostrils flared. Yet as I write this, I have just seen Farah on the Dave Letterman show, denying that she has ever had plastic surgery. What's the point? Is there *anybody* left in zip code 90210, Beverley Hills who has NOT had plastic surgery? Her nose looks terrible right now, which is tragic. She is one of my favourite beauties of all time and now, sadly, stands as an example of bad rather than good plastic surgery. To avoid this, while maintaining that youthful look, it is probably necessary to have one's face tweaked every two to three years by a (good) plastic surgeon.

This is where the allure of cosmetic surgery lies: you can get younger AND better-looking as you get older.

Well, plastic surgery younger…

Celebrity case-book

My publisher has asked me to do a round-up of the faces of people who appear regularly on the pages of magazines and newspapers in this country to illustrate what I am saying; although it will equally illustrate – as in the case of Farah – that not all do it successfully.

Some people – lawyers and celebrities mostly – might say that to discuss who has had what cosmetically enhanced is an invasion of privacy. Certainly, the majority of English people who voluntarily go under the scalpel prefer to keep it secret; they deny having had any surgery and attribute their everlasting youthful looks to healthy living, good genes and drinking lots of Evian. Others – such as Anne Robinson – have been candid on the subject of their transformation and have indeed made a virtue of it, but most of those who tell the truth are compelled to do so by such misfortune as a botched operation. Leslie Ash – of 'trout-pout' tabloid ridicule – is an example of this, but Mary Archer (wife of Jeffery) was only flushed out in the process of suing her embittered ex-personal assistant.

Yet is the law of privacy supposed to deny blatant reality? Everyone can see that certain people are defying the laws of nature, usually for a commercial motive; everyone knows that cosmetic surgery is behind it. Are we supposed to pretend that it's the 'youth-fairy' who is blessing them with ever-younger looks?

There are good and bad ways to deal with surgery, just as there is good and bad surgery. Joan Rivers not only looks fabulous for her age but also makes her resort to cosmetic surgery a very funny part of her act. On the other hand, Joan Collins forces newspapers that have reported her using cosmetic surgery, like the *Mail on Sunday* in 2002, to retract the allegation – and to apologise for 'any embarrassment caused'.

This cloud-cuckoo land hypocrisy is peculiarly English. Things are far more open and robust in America. American women swap names of plastic surgeons at lunch and compare the merits of their procedures with alacrity (and Farah Fawcett should join them, she'd feel better for it). Moreover, some (though thankfully not all) English journalists enjoy perpetuating the myth of film stars 'preserving' their looks or bodies and looking remarkably well in their dotage, seemingly without any intervention other than all that mineral water. These sycophantic columnists behave like medieval court troubadours singing their ladies' praises – immaculate ladies like Joan Collins, Felicity Kendal or Dame Judi Dench, who rather like Bernini's Teresa can never age. Even if the freedom of the press is so shackled that the English public cannot be told the truth, there is no excuse for writers to act like doting schoolboys – or Evian's PR team. Fortunately, the American press is not so rose-tinted in its view. They call a wrinkle a wrinkle and love to show the 'before' and 'after' photographs of their idols.

Anyway, here are some of my speculative observations on a number of well-known faces – and while photographs can lie they cannot lie that much.

Victoria Beckham

She has made the most of herself – you have to admire that. I think she's definitely had breast implants, despite her denials. If not, then they look like she has, which I mean as a compliment. She's had her lips injected. Her nose has been crimped – the tip has been made smaller and more defined. She's had Botox too – on her forehead.

UPSIDE: I think that she is a pretty girl, her nose is great. She has a petite body and wears clothes really well. She has good arms. Her eyes are small, but they are hazel, which is quite pretty, and have a nice shape to them. The lips were on the thin side in the early photographs, so she needed them done. She has great cheekbones. Somebody has told her or she figured it out by herself – as most people do eventually – what was required and she has gone and had it done.

DOWNSIDE: I think that unfortunately she is much too thin – which is really sad. I presume she is quite short and wears high heels as a lot of English women do – too high, in my view. Her eyebrows are quite low and don't do much for her. I would like to see her eyebrows more arched with an endoscopic brow lift. Her nasal tip needs to be made a little smaller and more defined. Her upper lip could be fuller with some Perlane or even better an Alloderm implant. Finally, we need some Botox between the eyebrows to keep that area smooth.

Joanna Lumley

At fifty-eight years old, work is unfortunately overdue. She needs a brow lift, a face-lift, eyelids (upper and lower), and a mid-face/cheek-lift to restore those famous cheekbones. All this followed by a full-face laser resurfacing.

Judi Dench

Is it legal to operate on Dames? I've operated on a few Ladies, but where I come from a *Dame* has a completely different meaning. Judi is overweight and desperately in need of losing that before she gets anything else done.

Michael Caine

Another messed up facelift – he looked dreadful for a long time and is just beginning to look human again. I don't think his wife Shakira has had anything done on the other hand. She is Indian and that race ages well – also, Indians are not usually in favour of cosmetic surgery. She is extremely beautiful, with high cheekbones – a woman like that can maintain her beauty well into her 60s.

Iman Bowie

Iman is another example: I don't find her particularly attractive, but she is ageing well too. Husband David just looks bizarre. Whatever caused his recent heart attack, though, it wasn't indulging in rhinoplasty.

Joan Collins

She's had enough work done. But I'd advise a different hair style, new colour and different outfits.

Mick Jagger

A face transplant, minus the lips.

Nicole Kidman

She has had her nose done and lost weight. She needs her upper lip done, it's too thin.

Owen Wilson

He should not have anything done to his nose. Like Stephen Fry's, it has become part of his character. It may look terrible, but without it he would be just another pretty-boy actor. Although the same cannot be said for Stephen… if he doesn't lose weight he'll soon look like Robert Morley.

Emma Thompson

No American actress would let herself be seen like this (*see photograph*). Sure, very few American actresses have a fraction of her acting ability – but she should wait until she has had her breasts done before attending openings without a bra. She needs a browlift. Her eyebrows are too low now and need to be lifted, and the muscle on her forehead needs to be smoothed out. She has too much extra skin on her upper eyelids, which needs to be trimmed, and far too many lines around the eyes. She needs some Botox and some laser re-surfacing of the skin. Plus she'll need a facelift and a lower necklift – and soon.

Jack Nicholson and Sean Connery

Neither has had anything done. Paul Newman, on the other hand had a facelift. Nicholson needs to lose weight, though Connery has got to be one of the best looking men on the planet and doesn't seem to mind being bald or somewhat overweight.

Robert Redford

Once credited with saying that he would never resort to cosmetic surgery, he has succumbed – the once-famous bags under the eyes have clearly gone in the latest photographs of him.

Mickey Rourke

His is a case of a terrible facelift. It's pulled his ears down and he looks odd. Paul Simon is another example of the same error. There's nothing I can recommend at this stage to help either of them.

Michael Douglas

A good-looking guy – one of the few men who have survived a facelift and looks better. Most men don't look good with facelifts: as well as Mickey Rourke, Paul Simon and Michael Caine, think of Burt Reynolds or Joe Pesci.

Cary Grant

In terms of a face model, he exemplified a great chin in a man. Cole Porter thought he was the best looking man alive and was delighted when Grant portrayed him in a film about his life. In the latest movie on Porter's life, *De-Lovely*, poor Kevin Kline cannot compare (although he does have a cleft chin).

Bill & Hilary Clinton

He's finally had the bags removed from his lower eyelids. Hilary has gotten older and prettier – got rid of the glasses and changed her hairstyle. She is still not the prettiest dame, however: she has piano legs, I'm afraid. For her I would recommend brow lift, upper and lower eye-lift and facelift, plus a skin program to improve her skin tones and quality.

Tony Blair

I do think he's kept in unusually good shape for a British politician. However, those youngish looks have become increasingly careworn and frayed recently. The ideal solution would be Botox to the frown lines and worry lines on the forehead, plus maybe a little tissue filler to the naso-labial lines from the angles of the mouth to the nose. And if he is feeling really adventurous, a course of three Isolagen treatments would ensure a more extensive make-over.

Julie Christie

She's had a facelift, of course. It looks OK, but she's lost a lot of hair, so it can't have been done very well. Her neck's not too good, either. This seems is a common problem in many of the neck-lifts I see in this country, usually caused by failure to deal with the muscles at the front of the neck called the platysmal bands.

Sophia Loren

She has had a lot done – several facelifts. In fact she's had surgery throughout her career. Her upper lip needs to be plumped up now. She is another star who pays tribute to Evian for her agelessness.

Ivana Trump

Her nose is beginning to droop a little bit. She had a great post-divorce coming out on the operating table, but now she has gained some weight and is due for another tune-up. The hair has to go. Soon they'll be calling her Carmen Miranda.

Sophie Dahl

She's had her lip plumped up, that much is certain. She's definitely had her nose done to go with her weight loss.

Elton John

He should get some of that fat off and consider a better hair transplant. Either that or just shave his head for a change.

Sam Taylor Wood

Her husband has my profound sympathy.

Jerry Hall

Personally I have never liked Jerry Hall, and never understood how she was such a successful model. There are many things about her I would fix if I had the chance. Her face has too many teeth and she is too tall, with a very high forehead. She now needs her frown lines and upper eyelids fixed. Her browlift is so badly done, she looks like she is prematurely balding. She needs a hair transplant because that forehead is unfeminine: she would look so much younger if she brought the hairline down. She's already had a facelift, which is too tight right now, but it will slacken down. I think she probably did it in the States, as it has the look of an American facelift. If she'd gone to a good plastic surgeon, he would have told her not to touch the brows – they have always been good. I would have just taken skin out of the upper eyelids, and never have done anything to the forehead, except some Botox. She needs to have her upper lip plumped up a bit more.

Her big problem is that she hasn't done the one thing she needed the most – her nose. She probably thinks 'the nose is me' and assumes that people associate her with this nose. While they probably do, it doesn't necessarily mean it suits her: in fact it makes her look sharp and hard. She needs her breasts lifted, too. And she should never, ever allow herself to be snapped in that position (*see photograph*).

Kylie Minogue

Her eyebrows remind me of Spock. It looks like she's had a 'temporal' face lift, and that the hairline has been pulled back above the ear along with the outer part of the eyebrow. I would also like to re-do her nose. She still has a great figure, though. She's had her lips plumped up and breast implants. Right now, what she needs is her upper eyelids done. She probably had her bum injected with fat, but I don't know what the big deal is about it – I've never been a great fan of her bum. Still, it clearly has its devotees – and she has great legs. Fat injections would lift the bum in any case, as long as one has fat to spare someplace else (which I don't think she has) – about 400 grams for both buttocks.

Jennifer Lopez

I would alter her hairstyle to something softer and get her out of short shorts. I'd like to Botox her forehead generally and bring her hair forward on either side of it, then narrow her nasal tip a little, if possible. Also, if she was really in the mood, hair transplants to lower her hair-line about one centimetre – which would make her look younger. This might be good after an eyebrow lift.

Heather Mills

On the downside, her teeth aren't very good – not by American standards. I personally don't find her attractive – her nose is too long and the nostrils are too wide when she smiles. She shows a bit too much gum and her nose comes down to meet her lip when she smiles. Her upper lip is too short – in fact I think both her lips are too thin. She has too many lines on her upper eyelids. I would recommend a brow-lift with an upper eyelid tuck and a laser resurfacing of her lower lids.

But overall physically she is not an unattractive woman – and what's most attractive about her is her spirit. This comes through in her face and underlines my point that beauty is made human by the way personality is reflected in the features. She has that sort of English look about her – she looks to me like someone who could be presenting *Blue Peter*. She is going to have that 'older mother syndrome' when her babies start school.

Jennifer Aniston

One of my favourites, but I would definitely still narrow the nasal bones. I would perk up the tip of the nose a little and make it smaller – plus a small chin implant.

Madonna

Ah, the Material Girl! An Italian-American from Detroit, Michigan, now forty-six years old. I think Madonna is a really difficult subject for me because despite her being enormously talented I have never personally found her attractive. I'd like to get her to a good orthodontist and a good cosmetic dentist – her teeth are just too much a part of her face. Her nose needs to be smaller and the tip higher. Again she needs an eyebrow lift. Her lips and mouth are too small. She has great cheeks, but then her eyes are too small. She's done a lot to keep her body fit, but if you look at her closely, she's got a thickish waist and heavy hips.

She would have had a facelift to get that almond shaped face. Her eyebrows have been trimmed. She's definitely had a nose job, because it was horrible before. Looking at some of the older photographs of her, she'd had her lips overdone on one, on another her eyebrows went all over the place, the skin quality is not very good and the blonde hair looked pretty awful. She never really seems to get it together, which is a shame.

Somebody with that much money should have someone tell her how to cut her hair. This is a hairstyle that does nothing for her (*see photograph*). Michelle Pfeiffer and Gwyneth Paltrow may have had this same style, but this kind of long blonde hair doesn't do anything for them either. And her dress sense is appalling.

Michelle Pfeiffer

Boy, she's just got better and better, hasn't she? She's had the works done: breasts, a facelift and browlift, and she had her nose tweaked and lips puffed up. It's that simple – she's a smart woman, her money is in her face and she has invested in it. It's a face worth investing in. You don't mess around with that kind of face, but you keep it looking good – unless you want to be out of business or are looking to retire.

Jordan

She is a sad case. Her breasts were quite pretty in the beginning and now they are an abomination – huge breasts, whether a personal decision or not, do tend to speak of a lack of sophistication and refinement. But if she likes them, well, that's what's important. She also has the English habit – lots of cover-up make-up. In fact Jordan epitomises the pleb look – and it's not just the English. Look at J-Lo, Kylie Minogue, Victoria Beckham and Joan Collins with their high heels, deep cleavage and short skirts – these are women who have money, but not much class. They are raunchy but too coarse. I don't say it to be cruel – it's just a fact. On the other hand, the ideal toff look is what you see in Tara Palmer Tomkinson: small breasts, slim hips, long legs, straight back – oh, and good posture from all that horse-riding. These are the qualities that separate the toffs from the plebs. That said, people can have class and it won't stop them being incredibly tedious and boring. And it still doesn't stop 99.9% of English males being completely agog at the sheer physics of Jordan's breasts.

Angelina Jolie

She doesn't need any work right now. As she got older, she got prettier. This is what happens when you learn how to do your hair up properly, start to dress well... oh, and have your lips injected and sharpen up your features. She's also lost 20 pounds, which she needed to lose. Does not need any work right now. This is a woman who's got somebody telling her how to dress. She should ring up Madonna and give her the name of her stylist. Her ex, Billy Bob Thornton, just had a facelift and a hair transplant and looks pretty good. I hope he gave Angelina her panties back and is once again wearing the trousers.

Sarah Jessica Parker

I like SJP. Here's another woman who's taken good advice on dressing. Her nose is, well... but it's her nose! She's had it tweaked but not enough to change it dramatically. I have grown to love it. She helps demonstrate how there is not one ideal of beauty. Her eyebrows are low, but she has great cheekbones – she has thin lips and a small mouth, yet she's still beautiful. And I happen to know that she is a delightful person. As you can tell, I am very much a fan of SJP. She's got style. And no woman should trade up her looks at the expense of her style.

Elizabeth Hurley

She is pretty, though her breasts have dropped a little over the years. I think she is beginning to look a bit old for this modelling lark. She's had her lips plumped up, that's for sure. A great set of teeth, but her eyes need doing.

Anne Robinson

She's traded that homely look for the ice-queen. She's had brow lift and a facelift. Her eyes were done but she still needs her lips made bigger. When I looked at her recently in the gameshow, post-facelift, she still had the two bands which stretch from the chin down to the base of the neck, which have clearly not been addressed (I suspect that is why she often wears a scarf). However, she has lost that homely look.

Susan Sarandon

She's just had a facelift – and she needed it. You may say it doesn't make her look like Susan Sarandon anymore, even if she does look nicer. But then, Susan Sarandon pre-surgery had stopped looking like her old self anyway. After a while you don't look like you used to – and so, you have to go and have a facelift. She did the wise thing.

Halle Berry

She has had the tip of her nose done. She has had a couple of operations to refine it, since it was a little bit too bulbous to start with.

Sharon Stone

Despite her ambivalence on the subject, she has most certainly had an excellent facelift quite recently (and adopted a much more flattering shorter haircut). If you compare her photographs from ten years ago, the face appears shorter and fuller now too – a dead giveaway of a facelift.

Ruby Wax

She resembles an unusually short truck driver…albeit one without muscle definition. If I had to work on her, I would prescribe liposuction of her abdomen, a facelift and neck-lift, artificial tan and softer skin colour – oh, and somehow add about 3 inches in height… Maybe on the rack…

Sven Goran Eriksson (…and his women)

Eriksson himself is obviously in good shape – toned and smartly dressed – and carries himself well. This, in combination with notoriety and deep pockets, has turned him into a target for women of a certain disposition. These include:

Ulrika Jonsson

I only know this lady from recent photographs. It is obvious that she was once quite cute, but like so many in this category, she is now resting on her past glory. Her breasts are sagging and her face needs everything done – facelift, fillers, Botox, the works.

Nancy Dell'Olio

A typical Italian – plumped up lips (most Italian women go for that look), and a curvaceous figure which is now thickening, making her trendy outfits look somewhat incongruous. Comparing photographs, she has obviously had a tummy tuck and breast implants. The face has been worked on, too. I wouldn't be surprised if she's had everything done, including her eyes tightened, a browlift, and – once again – facelift, fillers and Botox.

Faria Alam

Good dress sense, and a good figure with a small waist – clearly she's yet to fall pregnant. A very poor complexion, however – she needs to be on an intensive skin program.

ROYALTY:

Sarah Ferguson, Duchess of York

She's obviously had a facelift and she needed one when she had it done. She has a great set of teeth but her lips need plumping up desperately. She also needs some Botox – at least she did the last time I saw her. She probably needs some laser re-surfacing and another facelift.

In fact I'd like to get her on my operating table, I think she needs a bit of tightening up. She's had a chronic weight problem, which is very difficult to deal with. A brow lift at this point would correct her forehead issues.

Countess of Wessex

She is pretty and she knows how to dress, but the typical English pear-shape. She does have a bit of a big bum and her legs are a little thick. She has this sort of English-girl laugh where you open your mouth like it was some kind of flytrap and strain your eyes as if you are trying to look through a Venetian blind. In terms of her face, her nose needs to be softened; she has a beautiful jaw line, but her lips are a little thin. If she were in the movie business, I would suggest she get her lips plumped up and her nose softened. Her neck is a little thick and her breasts are probably on the small side, but that doesn't matter – look at who she married.

Duchess of Gloucester

I can just tell that she is a woman who needs help. She looks like she is wearing a military uniform (*see photograph*) – I don't know where the English sense of fashion comes from. It's amazing what outfits women wear in this country – some of them look like the drapes from stately homes. She obviously needs Botox and a good skin program. She needs an eye job and a facelift, and she's hiding her neck by wearing this scarf. Actually this is a classic English hairdo dating from the mid-16th century, which fortunately we have royalty to keep in fashion – otherwise nobody else would do it. This is one of the few tasks left for the royalty, to maintain arcane styles of dress and coiffure.

The Queen

At 78 she is a bit of an anachronism, really – a sweet old lady who is out of shape and wears incredibly awful coats and hats.

Thankfully they cover up what promises to be a terrifying body underneath. She would see better if she did her upper eyelids. Otherwise leave well alone. No-one can look very good with a tiara and that hair-do.

There is a huge chasm between the First Lady in the US and the Brits' equivalent. The former, usually with no experience, invariably carry it off. The Royals – who must have been practicing their dress and manners since the time of William the Conqueror – are more often than not just *off.*

Camilla Parker Bowles

I gather that she is a lovely woman and a lot of fun to be with, and that's probably the most important thing about her (or, for that matter, anybody). Beyond than that there is really nothing positive I can say, not about her appearance. She needs upper and lower eyelid blepharoplasty, brow lift, facelift, chin implant and a smaller, more feminine nose – followed by a full-face laser resurfacing. But if she is comfortable with how she looks and doesn't want to do anything, then she shouldn't.

We should never forget to look at the whole person. There are some horribly, horribly superficial people out there who may have a surface beauty – like a very delicate doll or a mannequin – and one that we might casually admire. But there is absolutely no point in standing next to them at a party and trying to hold a conversation as there is nothing to talk about. I am sure that after ten minutes talking to Camilla, you would become oblivious to her appearance.

She has made the most of herself – you have to admire that. I think she's definitely had breast implants, despite her denials. If not, then they look like she has, which I mean as a compliment. She's had her lips injected. Her nose has been crimped – the tip has been made smaller and more defined. She's had Botox too – on her forehead.

Not a lot of people know this but she was called Posh because her father used to pick her up from school in a Bentley.

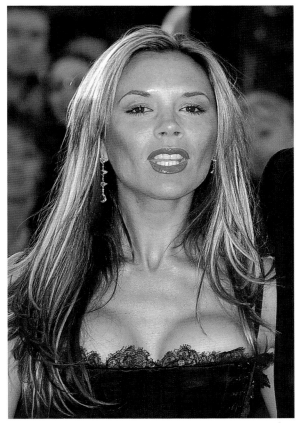

Victoria Beckham 2004 [XWF]

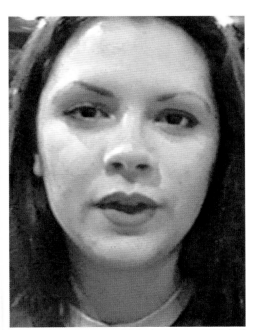

Victoria Adams 2001 [ZZ]

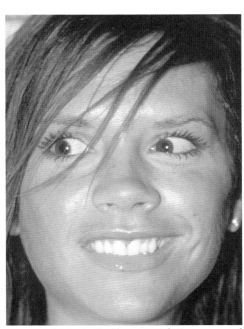

Victoria Beckham2001 [Nils Jorgensen]

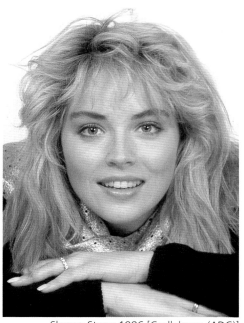

Sharon Stone 1986 [Crollalanza (ADC)]

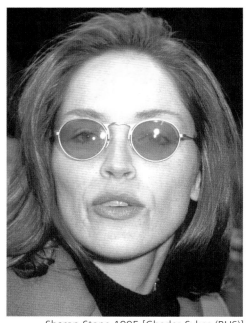

Sharon Stone 1995 [Charles Sykes (RUS)]

Despite Sharon Stone's ambivalence on the subject, she has most certainly had an excellent facelift quite recently (and adopted a much more flattering shorter haircut). If you compare her photographs from ten years ago, the face appears shorter and fuller now too – a dead giveaway of a facelift. Plus her hairline is travelling back across her head, ergo the hairdo.

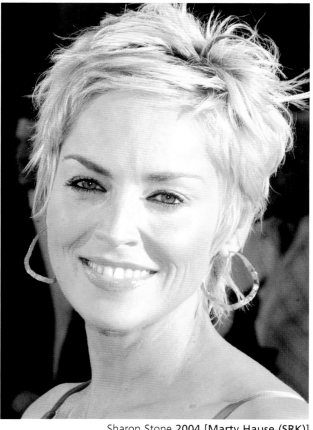

Sharon Stone **2004** [Marty Hause (SRK)]

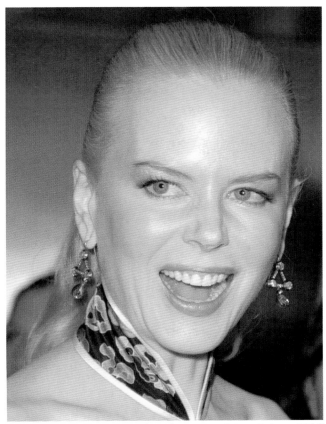

She has had her nose done and lost weight. She needs her upper lip done, it's too thin. Even though pictures often lie, there is a limit. And these pictures speak for themselves.

Nicole Kidman **2004 [Matt Beirne BBN]**

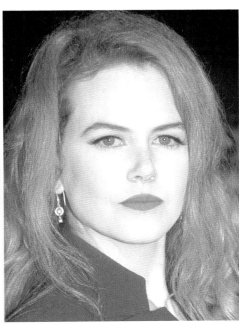

Nicole Kidman 1992 [Rex, Randy Bauer A/C

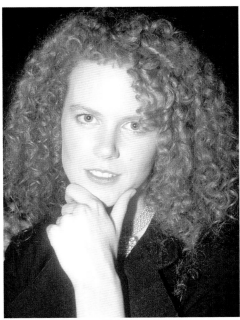

Nicole Kidman 1989 [Brendan Beirne (BBN)]

Her browlift is so badly done, she looks like she is prematurely balding. She needs a hair transplant because that forehead is unfeminine: she would look so much younger if she brought the hairline down. She's already had a facelift, which is too tight right now, but it will slacken down. I think she probably did it in the States, as it has the look of an American facelift. If she'd gone to a good plastic surgeon, he would have told her not to touch the brows – they have always been good. I would have just taken skin out of the upper eyelids, and never have done anything to the forehead, except some Botox. She needs to have her upper lip plumped up a bit more.

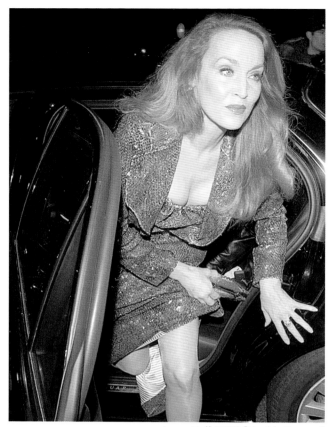

Jerry Hall 2004 [Huckle/Jaguar]

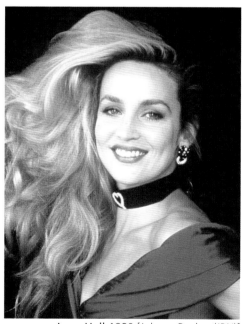

Jerry Hall 1990 [Johnny Boylan (JBN)]

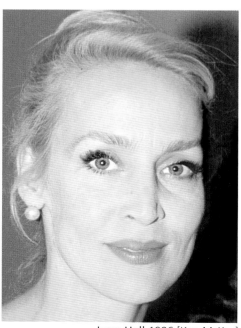

Jerry Hall 1996 [Ken McKay]

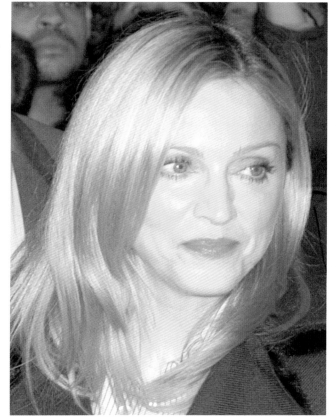

She would have had a facelift to get that almond shaped face. Her eyebrows have been trimmed. She's definitely had a nose job, because it was horrible before. Looking at some of the older photographs of her, she'd had her lips overdone on one, on another her eyebrows went all over the place, the skin quality is not very good and the blonde hair looked pretty awful. She never really seems to get it together, which is a shame.

Madonna 2003 [DH/Keystone USA]

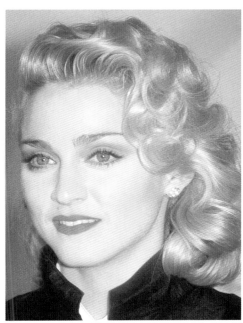

Madonna 1986 [Herbie Knott]

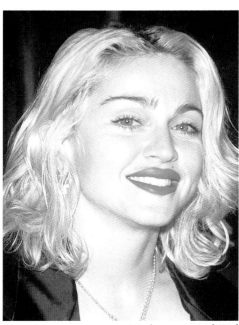

Madonna 1984 [KBU]

Boy, she's just got better and better, hasn't she? She's had the works done: breasts, a facelift and browlift, and she had her nose tweaked and lips puffed up. It's that simple – she's a smart woman, her money is in her face and she has invested in it. It's a face worth investing in. You don't mess around with that kind of face, but you keep it looking good – unless you want to be out of business or are looking to retire.

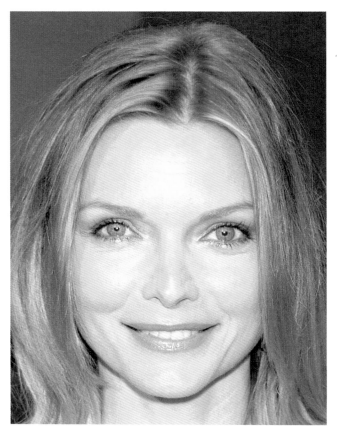

Michelle Pfeiffer **2003** [UMDADC (ADC)]

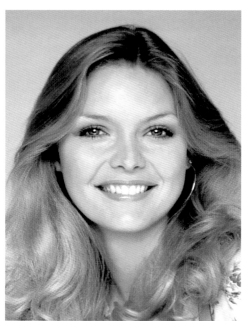

Michelle Pfeiffer 1979 [Everett Collection (EVT)]

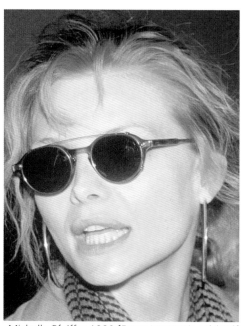

Michelle Pfeiffer 1989 [Fotos International (FIN)]

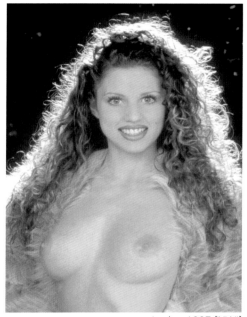

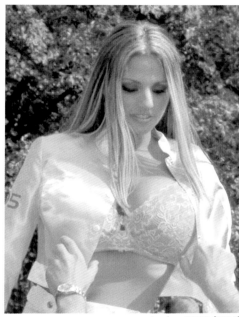

Jordan 1997 [NWI]

Jordan 2004 [NWI]

She is a sad case. Her breasts were quite pretty in the beginning and now they are an abomination... they do tend to speak of a lack of sophistication and refinement. Jordan epitomises the pleb look – and it's not just the English. Look at J-Lo, Kylie Minogue, Victoria Beckham and Joan Collins with women who have money, but not much class. They are raunchy but too coarse.

The Duchess has obviously had a facelift and she needed one when she had it done.

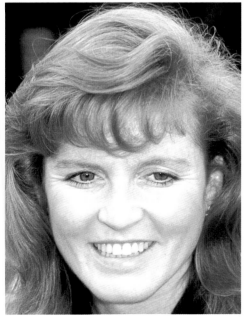

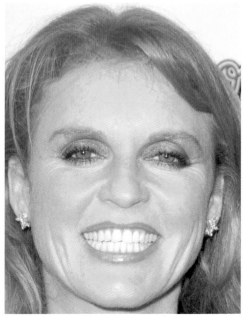

Sarah Ferguson 1991 [Nils Jorgensen (NJ)]   Sarah Ferguson 2004 [Matt Baron/BEI]

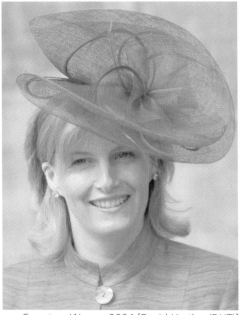

Countess Wessex 2004 [David Hartley (DHT)]

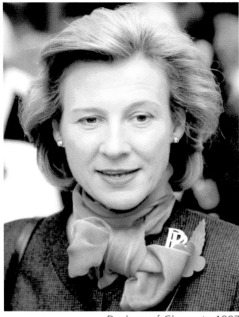

Duchess of Gloucester1997
[South Coast Press (SCP)]

The Countess's neck is a little thick and her breasts are probably on the small side, but that doesn't matter – look at who she married.   I can just tell that the Duchess is a woman who needs help. She looks like she is wearing a military uniform.

Charles is gangly and his eyes are set too closely together. Unfortunately only a cranio-facial surgeon could correct this. He looks like he's already had a hair transplant, and his ears were pinned back.

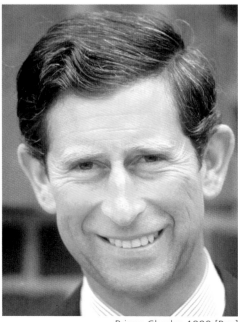

Prince Charles 1990 [Rex]

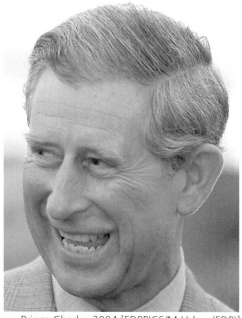

Prince Charles 2004 [EDPPICS/M Usher (EDP)]

Prince Charles

He is gangly and his eyes are set too closely together. Unfortunately only a cranio-facial surgeon could correct this. He looks like he's already had a hair transplant, and his ears were pinned back. His complexion is awful. As a physical specimen, there is no hope.

He is a man who knows how to dress, however. He does wear nice suits and I love his shirts and some of his ties. But does he have to put a handkerchief in his top pocket? It just looks foppish. And the more narrow ties are very English – they look silly. I wish he'd take his hands out of his pockets - also a very English disease which I detest. I suppose it's better than pocket billiards, but it ruins the way the jacket hangs. It is sort of a pose that a physician takes when he has a white coat on. It reminds me of those *Doctor in the House* movies with Hattie Jacques as Matron and James Robertson Justice as the Consultant Surgeon standing authoritatively at the end of the bed. I think Charles and I must have watched the same old movies.

When you are a Royal nobody cares whether you are handsome or not – it's the title they're interested in. I personally think of them as just another kind of pop star. I treat all of my celebs the same way as my other patients, except in one way (*see* – Surgeon's Fees). If you allow yourself to treat them differently, I think ultimately it prevents you taking good care of them as a physician. If they are the kind of celebrity who can't bear to be treated like an ordinary mortal, then it is best they consult my competitors.

Most of my celebrity patients are very easy to deal with. Titled patients seem mainly interested in talking about which football team I support! The answer is none.

The actors and actresses enjoy being treated normally, and I love to talk to them about their work – but I don't let it get in the way of mine. Seeing them on stage or in a movie makes me appreciate their talent from a different perspective as I observe the transformation from 'patient' to 'star'.

I feel a twinge of sadness when I look at Michael Jackson today – I recall first meeting him in 1983, when he looked quite normal and I was a plastic surgery trainee at the University of Southern California. I was moonlighting as an Emergency Room doctor at Encino Hospital in the San Fernando Valley, and one evening Michael Jackson walked in with his nephew who had fallen off the 'Stage' at home where they were putting on a show. I stitched up the cut on the nephew's forehead and told Michael that I was a trainee Plastic Surgeon. This didn't seem to interest him in the least. Rumour has it that in later years, plastic surgeons would sedate him and pretend to operate on him – because that was the only way to deal with his addiction to plastic surgery.

The hidden price
Very few people are naturally beautiful. Most people have to work at it – whether they use make-up, clothes or cosmetic surgery.

Those who don't, try to play up the good parts and disguise the bad ones. But they are all seeking an aesthetic ideal.

On the other hand, an unlimited amount of money and willingness to submit to the knife will not necessarily turn a person into a fabulous beauty, although it will definitely help. Michael Jackson is a perfect illustration of the above, though his case is so media-exposed it scarcely needs exhuming here.

It is a sad fact of life that an unlimited amount of money often leads to unlimited amounts of surgery, without making the end results attractive. Consider super-wealthy people such as Jackson, or Jocelyn Wildenstein (the so called 'cat woman' of New York). Observe also Mary Tyler Moore, Joan Rivers and numerous others who have had their surgical excesses well-documented in the press. There are patients of mine with whom money is not an issue, and yet I see in them lots of complications resulting from repetitive and bad surgery (by other surgeons, of course). There occasionally comes a point when I tell my patients, 'You are the best that I can make you. I can make you worse, but I can't make you better.' Or to put it another way, *the enemy of good is better*.

Not every surgeon is as forthright, and one should beware of surgeons capitalising on patients' insecurities. More money will not always buy the best results. Some plastic surgeons will charge based solely on the patients' ability to spend. It is only plastic surgeons who go to Saudi Arabia, for example, to do a single procedure who can and do charge totally disproportionately – a little like a famous Western singer performing privately for a rich Sultan. An appropriate fee for going to a country where the outcome of surgery can be contentious is close to $100,000 minimum.

Inflated fees notwithstanding, Middle Eastern women are great consumers of not only designer clothing, but plastic surgery too. We have seen an increase in the number of people in the Middle East who have been converted to cosmetic surgery. They spend a tremendous amount on enhancing their appearance, because even though they may not be subject to the same peer pressure that motivates their West European counterparts, female company is still greatly competitive – and they feel an additional need to try harder to please their husbands and psych out their rivals.

Image enhancement
While plastic surgery can change the person, computer software can digitally alter the photographic image, using a computer screen as a virtual operating theatre. Today, we can enhance the appearance of female beauty on two levels: surgically improving the initial subject matter, and then if necessary 'touching up' the secondary image – that is, the photo.

People are just not aware of the way images are manipulated by the media. A prime example of this is the magazine cover of Kate Winslet, when the elongated, thinned-out body that hit news-stands shocked even the actress herself.

Every image – and I would like to emphasise this – *every* image that goes on the cover of a magazine is digitally enhanced. The majority of photographs taken today are digital and can be uploaded onto a computer immediately. These pictures are re-framed so that an editor can go through a huge selection of them and pick the one that works best. The angle at which the photograph is taken can accentuate one feature over another. The selection then goes through different stages of improvement.

Usually, the first thing that is done is the softening of the shadows to smooth out the skin complexion. The colour of the skin and consistency of the complexion are then improved: wrinkles are airbrushed and lines are smoothed (every model does have lines – but they can be airbrushed out). The jaw line may be sharpened. Yet these are just the subtle things. The major 'surgery' affects the figure: waists can be tightened, legs elongated, and so on.

The image of beauty itself moves with the flavour of the month – what's the best nose, what are the best eyes? Even if the nose or eyes are not the right flavour, they can be changed to ensure that they are on the cover.

Beauty is on the cusp of changing more radically than ever before – and more rapidly, too. We are not going to see static images of beauty anymore. Individuals are going to change, but in the process they are going to become more stereotyped – and what people perceive as the ideal is going to become ever more consistent.

In theory now every woman is going to want to have a small nose, for instance, and no one is going to have a big nose. And everyone is going to want to have big lips and no one is going to have small lips. In fact everyone is going to want to look the same at the same time. Beauties that exist outside of our accepted stereotypes, such as Anjelica Huston, may be no more.

We will not see the range of beauty that we may have seen in the past – and that is rather sad.

The Plastic Surgery Code [PSC]:
(Its application to the the different stages of ageing)

There is, in fact, a certain plastic surgery code evolving. Everybody always covets a particular 'must-have' facial feature – a good example of this is the type of nose that in the 70s and 80s became the trademark of a New York surgeon, Howard Diamond. This type of nose was and still is referred to as 'the Diamond nose'. Dr. Diamond was an Ear Nose and Throat surgeon, now retired, who did a total of 14,000 noses in his career, beginning in the 1960s and ending in the mid-1990s. Jacques Joseph did a roaring trade in the 30s making Jewish noses look smaller because there was so much anti-semitism.

People aspire to social conformity from an early age. If you look at teenagers, mostly they dress the same, talk with the same high pitched voice and jabber on their cell phones simultaneously. The trend is to belong to a group and that includes being thin, having a cute nose and yes, cute breasts and a cute butt. If you haven't got it, you try to acquire it. Noses are increasingly remodelled in adolescence and there is a distinction between children whose parents who can afford to have it done and those who have to wait till adulthood and pay for it themselves.

The same applies to orthodontics. A number of adult people are now walking around with braces on the teeth, because they may be wealthy now but weren't wealthy as kids. Good quality teeth are a part of the plastic surgery code – they need to be well maintained and they need to have a good colour (they shouldn't be yellow, and certainly not brown). Also the edges ought to be even. There are subtleties only a trained eye would spot, but if you look like Dracula, it's clear you won't have spent much time in a cosmetic dentist's surgery. Good teeth are considered even more important in the US where even small gaps between the teeth are taken care of in childhood.

The other thing that women look at in adolescence is breasts. If they don't have breasts then they want breast augmentation and again, what it boils down to is whether the parents can pay for this early on or whether the child has to bide her time. It may sound like a horror story, but in Texas it is not uncommon to give a breast augmentation to a 16-year-old as her birthday present. Certainly even with parental consent this would be an absolute minimum in my book. Eighteen is the age of majority in the States, and in the code of practice observed by the American Society of Plastic Surgeons this is recommended as a minimum age for breast augmentation.

You don't want to have enormous breasts – but then no breasts at all is not part of the PSC practice. The shape of the thighs definitely is a part of the PSC – if you have either violin or cello deformity of the thighs, that's correctable with surgery and at a younger age one would have liposculpture to eradicate this problem. In a very young group, you are not looking at Botox yet, but you are definitely looking at lip augmentation. If you have very thin lips you could have them plumped up with Perlane.

So, even in adolescence, teens and twenties, there is a lot that can be done to give people a helping hand.

And if you look at the next age group – late 20s to early 30s – we see people who have really taken care of themselves. This means not only going to the spa, but having some Botox and lip plumping. Throw in lifestyle considerations like working out at the gym, not smoking or sun-worshipping, and drinking moderate amounts of alcohol, then these people are easily distinguishable from the rest.

However, this generation does need to be especially mindful of the damage sun exposure can cause to the skin. Otherwise they will pay the price the previous, less well-informed generation paid – photoageing. The British are particularly prone to this since they do not possess the olive complexion of, say, South Americans (whose skin performs a little better under the sun). Smoking also damages the skin, something teenagers are not properly aware of when they start lifetime habits that will prematurely age them.

The next age group I would define as mid to late 30s. People in that group who have had short scar facelifts will look as good as they did in their early 20s, and that will definitely mark them apart. They will look great for the next 15 years and they will definitely look better than people who wait an extra 10 to 15 years to have a facelift. Provided they've had a good operation and chosen their surgeon carefully rather than spontaneously, these people are sure to age better than those who start later in life. This group will also be ideal for an isolated cheek lift because, as yet they don't have the extra skin.

If one is comfortable looking their age, then that is fine. But there is a group of women in the public eye who personify agelessness – women such as Nancy Reagan and Jackie Kennedy. In this country, say, the Duchess of Kent, Diana Rigg and Julie Andrews have obviously adhered to the PSC.

If a woman over 50 does look her age, then for whatever reason she hasn't observed the code. Some people age better than others and don't need surgery (I know women in their 70s who look remarkable) but we are talking about percentages here. So, the average woman should have had her eyelids done at about 40. Coming up to 50 nowadays is almost too late for a facelift. The results are going to be less natural. Certainly, at that age, the eyes have to be addressed – the eyelid should be tight not wrinkly, there should be no bags under the eyes or extra skin on the upper eyelid, and the eyebrows should have a nice arch. That is why the endoscopic browlift at a younger age is a very good procedure: it lifts the brows and the upper eyelid, so more and more commonly this technique is combined with eyelid surgery on a frequent basis.

The message is: *it's better to start earlier rather than later for the result to look more natural.*

I NEED IT **NOW**!

The essential procedures

How to choose a plastic surgeon

A plastic surgeon's training is usually founded upon extensive practice in general surgery. This means that he is conversant with all parts of the body from the top of the head to the tips of the toes, and that he has many years of surgical experience. This way, if patients have any complications at all, he can be confident in managing them. This also means he has a good professional relationship with his colleagues and can call upon a suitable physician to help avert any problems that might occur if surgery were contemplated – for instance, having a lung doctor examine someone who has a history of asthma; which is the preferred course of action.

In America, the distinction is fairly clearly cut as to who is well-trained. The training involves 5 years of general surgery and 2-3 years of plastic surgery, followed by one year in a specialised area such as cosmetic surgery. After this they would be in practice and certified by the American Board of Plastic Surgery. Once they have established themselves in practice and demonstrated that they have expertise in cosmetic plastic surgery, which usually takes several years, they can become a member of the American Society for Aesthetic Plastic Surgery (ASAPS). A member of ASAPS must do at least seventy-five cosmetic cases every year.

So, if shopping in the US, I would definitely recommend an ASAPS member. In England it is less clear-cut. There is no real effort to disseminate relevant information. There is generally a lack of organised training in cosmetic plastic surgery.

English practitioners are always surprised that it takes only 3 years to train a US counterpart, whereas it take 7 years to train in plastic surgery in this country. The reason is that when you start your cosmetic surgery training in the United States, you are already a trained general surgeon. Equally you know that you really have to use the next 3 years in a concentrated manner, because after that you will be in independent practice. You are aware that when you finish training you will be a practising surgeon, most frequently on your own– whereas in England, when you finish your training there is no guarantee that you will become a consultant.

There is, nonetheless, a body of cosmetic plastic surgeons in the UK who belong to the British Association of Aesthetic Plastic Surgeons

(BAAPS). They are self-described as the gold standard, however, it has to be understood that this is in reference to the UK only.

There are many other societies of cosmetic surgeons here and in different countries, and certainly many distinguished foreign plastic surgeons who do not belong to BAAPS. They're none-the-less at the very top of their profession and without a doubt gold standard in and of themselves. Ivo Pitanguy of Brazil and Yves-Gérard Illouz of France, Marco Gasparotti of Rome among many, many others. So, another criterion to look at is whether a surgeon belongs to an international society of cosmetic plastic surgeons such as the International Society of Aesthetic Plastic Surgery (ISAPS) to which BAAPS and ASAPS members belong.

In this day and age, there are more and more American plastic surgeons that travel to Europe on a regular basis to perform procedures, so distance should not be a criterion or a practical consideration when choosing a practitioner.

Lastly, all things being equal, personality should be taken into consideration, because if a level of communication cannot be established between patient and surgeon, then their relationship should be a short-lived one. A patient is entitled to having their questions answered, and a surgeon should not be allowed to suggest a procedure without explaining how it would benefit the patient. A surgeon should be able to provide information on how many operations they have done, and offer 'before and after' pictures – a good range of them.

Of course, if the surgeon is known by reputation it may be unnecessary to ask for these pictures. Patients can ask too many questions and if they have been 'shopping around' a surgeon might reasonably assume that they are not serious about having surgery, but are indulging in price comparison and window shopping.

Asking questions about post-surgery diet, exercise and garments-to-wear after surgery is wasting a surgeon's time during consultation, because the answers can be obtained in the lead time before the operation, during a second consultation or at the time of the procedure or even on a surgeon's website. I keep all of my instructional sheets and consent forms in a down-loadable form on my web site. The consultation is solely to determine what type of procedures are suitable for a patient and typically lasts half an hour. The exception to this is my vein consultation when I spend an hour explaining how veins work and why injection therapy is the treatment of choice.

The same applies to asking questions about malpractice suits of which every surgeon has a few, particularly in the United States which is so prone to legal recourse. If a new patient opens the conversation by asking that, a surgeon would be disinclined to take them on because no one likes litigious customers.

In fact, a consultation is very much a two-way interview and a surgeon may turn a new patient down on a variety of grounds, not least because they might not require any surgery at that particular moment. Despite the importance of not leaving things too late, Sir Harold Gillie's adage 'Don't do today what you can do tomorrow' is one all cosmetic surgeons should remember. I prefer to take the long term view and tell a patient to come and see me in 2 years time when I feel this would be to their benefit.

My own leitmotif is 'for the difference to be a difference, one must make a difference'. If a patient has made a decision to have cosmetic surgery, they are entitled to expect a difference that is a tangible improvement. The risk/reward ratio should still be in favour of the reward. No-one wants to go through the surgery, the recuperation period and the expense for a minimal result or obviously a worse result than they started with..

Great plastic surgeons are those who have created a new paradigm, a new era and a new way of thinking.

Ivo Pitanguy, is possibly the best known cosmetic plastic surgeon on the planet. What made him famous is his ability to teach as a well as operate – he has an institute of cosmetic surgery that is visited by many surgeons. Then, there is Marco Gasparotti in Rome who has done a great deal of innovative work in the area of liposuction.

Here it is also worth mentioning the likes of Jack Sheen, Jacques Joseph and Gustave Aufricht. There are hundreds of great surgeons, alive and dead who have advanced the art and science of plastic surgery.

Jacques Joseph suffered an ignominious end at the hands of the Nazis when they gave him an 'exit interview' before his proposed emigration to the United States in 1934. Gustave Aufricht, a fellow plastic surgeon, had arranged for Joseph to go and practice in New York City, where he would have been a great success. Joseph, however, never made it through the interview, which was a great loss to plastic surgery.

When I was in Australia and first became interested in PS, a surgeon named Bill Wilson, who was a Catholic and a great influence on me, once told me that, 'The Jews don't have the manual dexterity to be good plastic surgeons.' I was far too afraid to tell him that I was myself of Jewish descent, and worried for the greatest possible time that I could never be a plastic surgeon because I didn't have the required dexterity. I did briefly wonder whether I should perhaps convert to Catholicism… This anecdote now seems somewhat ironic, because the majority of plastic surgeons in LA are Jewish – although in Manhattan there is still a resistance to having Jewish plastic surgeons on staff at some hospitals.

Non-surgical procedures:

(road-side assistance from skin creams to acids and beyond)

As we get older, surgery may not be the first thing we should consider – rather, we may wish to maintain our looks by way of non-surgical treatments. For some patients this is preferable both medically and economically.

There are basically two types of non-surgical beauty procedures: a skin program is one, injections are another. Before we consider injectables, we need to consider our skin quality and invest in a good program. There are three problems that any skin program should address:

Pigmentation, fine or deep lines or wrinkles, and breakouts.
Pigmentation is usually managed with Hydroquinone, a bleaching agent, and Wrinkles and Acne are treated initially with Tretinoin and chemical peels. Acne can also be helped with antibiotics applied to the skin as well as Isotretinoin oral therapy for severe acne.

The skin is composed of three layers from above down, the epidermis with a layer of dead cells on top known as the stratum corneum, the dermis below the epidermis which contains a papillary layer containing a network of small blood vessels called capillaries and a reticular layer (containing the collagen fibres which give the skin its thickness) and lastly the subcutaneous layer containing a layer of fat with which we are all too familiar. In time, we suffer a loss of our youthful complexion due to the build up of the layer of dead cells on the surface of the skin. This is a normal part of our skin which becomes thicker with age representing the thin keratinized cells on the surface of the skin which are naturally exfoliated. The build up of this layer is exacerbated by applying facial moisturisers and foundation.

Moisturisers and foundation are the greatest myths of modern day skin care.

Exploding consumer myths

Self-application face creams are a hugely lucrative industry that trades upon the average consumer's lack of understanding of basic dermatology (which is the science of skin).

For all practical purposes, there is no face or eye cream on the retail market that is better than the next one. Thus, Crème de la Mer is no better in terms of repairing the skin than, say, Nivea cream. It is mainly a question of marketing. Despite decades of use by the majority of the population .Most women see no obvious improvement in their skin or prevention of ageing through the use of these products.

Even worse is that by applying foundation and moisturiser we are preventing the skin from exfoliating naturally and thus increasing its thickness. This in turn obscures the underlying colour of blood in the capillaries in the part of the skin known as the papillary dermis. (*see* http://travel.howstuffworks.com/sunscreen)

The oxygenated blood in our capillaries gives us a pink, healthy glow. The best way to moisturise the skin is to drink lots of fluid, preferably water. Healthy skin will then moisturise itself.

Circumstances that do require the application of moisturisers include extreme weather conditions (such as sub-zero temperatures) or excessive dryness. Maintaining a high intake of water, a regular exercise routine and a sensible skin care program would give one a much better complexion than the use of any hyped-up cream or foundation. One's basic skin care should include the use of a cleanser, a toner and a good exfoliating agent – and exclude the application of moisturisers on a routine basis I think of moisturizers as the junk food of our skin care program just as French-fries are the junk in our diet.

Sunscreen

Sunlight arrives on earth in three forms: infrared (heat), visible light and ultraviolet. Ultraviolet light is classified into three categories:

UVA (315 to 400 nm), also known as black light, which causes tanning

UVB (280 to 315 nm), which causes damage in the form of sunburn

UVC (100 to 280 nm), which is filtered out by the atmosphere and never reaches us.

Ninety-nine percent of the sun's UV radiation at sea level is UVA. It is the UVB that causes most of the problems related to sun exposure: things like aging, wrinkles, cancer and so on, although research is increasingly implicating UVA as well.

One of the interesting things about UV radiation is that it is reflected by different surfaces. These reflections can amplify the effects of UV exposure. For example, snow reflects 90% of UV light. That is why you can get snow blindness and severe sunburns from skiing on a sunny day. Sand can reflect up to 20% of UVB that hits it, meaning that you can get extra UV exposure at the beach.

On the other hand, certain things absorb almost all UV radiation partially or completely. Glass is one of these substances - many glasses are very good absorbers of UV (which is why you may have heard that you cannot get sunburn in a greenhouse - just make sure it is glass and not plastic covering the greenhouse!). Most sunscreens use chemicals that have the same UV-absorbing properties. (*see* http://travel.howstuffworks.com/sunscreen)

Exposure to ultraviolet light, UVA or UVB, from sunlight accounts for 90% of the symptoms of premature skin aging. Most of the photoaging effects occur by age 20. The amount of damage to the skin caused by the sun is determined by the total lifetime amount of radiation exposure and the person's pigment protection.

Sunscreen, is critical. If you avoid sun damage, you essentially avoid a lot of the problems associated with ageing. Sun damage causes thinning of the collagen layers of the skin. More crucially, it causes the elastin in the skin to lose its cross-linkages, removing the supporting structure of the skin. This is one of the main reasons why we have sagging of the facial and body tissues, other than gravity itself (if we walked upside down our entire life, we would actually age in the opposite direction – an interesting thought!).

Choosing the right sunscreen is absolutely essential. Any SPF product should be 'micronised', meaning it contains very small particles which can penetrate deeply into the skin. Micronised products are clear rather than white when applied.

The best sun blocks now have zinc and titanium in them for complete protection. Sun blocks should be SPF 30 or greater and they should be applied on a regular basis throughout the day – every few hours. Start thirty minutes before you step outside. If you are in the sun, it doesn't matter how high the sun protection, you still have to re-apply it. If you go in the water, you need a waterproof sun screen. These are basic points but people still forget. Driving in a car still requires sun-block and cloudy days do not prevent the ultra-violet radiation from damaging your skin. Remember: The ideal sunscreen has a micronised zinc and titanium oxide for broad spectrum UV-A protection. The chemical sunscreens (methoxycinnamate and octyl salicylate) boost the SPF level to help provide good UV-B protection. I recommend Elta Blocks (again no financial interest) which are PABA-free and safe for the sensitive skin. Elta Block SPF 32 uses a combination block & light moisturizer base for daily use on face, hands and arms. This product is excellent for use under makeup. Use in conjunction with Retin-A therapy, with photosensitive medications, and after plastic surgery.

Effective solutions – a skin program is the first step

Tretinoin (Retin-A, Avita, Renova) is a derivative of Vitamin A and is the treatment of choice for comedonal acne, or whiteheads and blackheads. It works by increasing skin cell turnover promoting the extrusion of the plugged material in the follicle. It also prevents the formation of new comedones. Tretinoin is also the only topical medication that has been proven to improve wrinkles.

Side Effects of Retin-A

The effect of increased skin cell turnover can be irritation and flaking. For this reason, many people stop using Retin-A after a couple of days to weeks, then think that it didn't work. It is important to realize that Retin-A is very effective for whiteheads and blackheads, but it may take 6-9 weeks to see a noticeable difference.

One should approach skin problems by first correcting the pigmentation flaws and trying to thicken the collagen layer, while also trying to thin the external stratum corneum layer of the skin. We can thin the external layer with Tretinoin to increase cell turnover. Tretinoin will also cause the collagen layer to thicken. Tretinoin is only available on prescription – there are some non-prescription derivatives available now, but tretinoin is what plastic surgeons and dermatologists normally use. It is often combined with a bleaching cream, such as Hydroquinone, to improve any abnormal pigmentation.

Tretinoin dries the skin initially – but continued use results in the skin acclimatising itself and the quality of it improving vastly. A lot of people who try Tretinoin find it doesn't work, because they don't use it for long enough or only apply it to small spots on their face. It should also be used as part of a co-coordinated skin program. A typical scenario is a patient obtaining a doctor's prescription for Tretinoin and beginning to use it by dabbing a little on at night. After a while, they see some crusting and peeling of the skin and call their doctor who advises that they should use a lesser amount or stop the application altogether because he does not understand that this is a desirable response

Tretinoin has to be applied evenly on the face. It is supposed to produce redness and burning, peeling and crusting (if you read the package it will tell you so), and this is in fact a therapeutic response. The discomfort normally lasts for about 6 weeks, and if you continue to use it, the reaction calms down – yet the Tretinoin is still doing its job.

Tretinoin can be used both in the morning and at night. Most often I recommend a nightly application because of the sun-sensitising effects of the medication. Its effects on the face are un-even because the thickness and character of our facial skin changes depending on the part of the face.. The forehead is thick scalp skin and, as such, very resistant to Tretinoin – as is the skin on the nose and the central part of the face. Eyelid skin is the thinnest in the body and such is very sensitive areas as are the outer parts of the cheeks, plus the angles of the mouth and the neck. The neck is more sensitive because it lacks a many of the oil glands in the face, so that dryness and burning is more likely to occur. Thus, you will see more of a response in some areas and less in others. In the forehead area and the usually oily "T" or central area of the face you have to apply more Tretinoin.

Normally, a plastic surgeon would put patients on a Tretinoin program at night but, if a more aggressive approach is adopted, the morning application is added. A patient who has oily skin is going to tolerate Tretinoin better than a patient with a dry skin. Tretinoin dries the skin so an oily skin will tolerate a more aggressive treatment where a dry skin will become more irritated and sensitive. Those with oily skin also need a much more intense program because first of all they need to get rid of that oiliness, which in turn reduces their breakouts and their acne if they have it. (*see* http://dermatology.about.com/cs/topicals/a/tretinoin)

Getting the full Monty – starts with a good skin program and it takes time
There is no quick fix in terms of getting flawless skin.
Anyone who wants to have a beautiful and healthy skin would need to go see a dermatologist or a plastic surgeon and adopt a skin care program that incorporates all of the elements above.

The essentials of any medical skin program are a cleanser and a toner morning and night. Hydroquinone is also applied under a sun-screen in the morning followed by the use of Tretinoin and Hydroquinone together before bed-time. A sun block is used during the day.

A good skin program requires three cycles of 6 weeks each to achieve the optimum result. A skin cycle consists of 6 weeks because that is the length of time it takes for a skin cell to go from the bottom layer of the epidermis to the top layer (magazine advertisements promising that you can look good in three weeks are nonsense, because the skin cannot re-cycle itself in less than six weeks). We refer to the first cycle as the 'I hate it' phase because that is when the burning and the 'bad' effects of tretinoin occur. Still, a lot of people don't mind that and are quite happy to go out looking that way.

The middle phase is the 'I like it' phase – that's the next 6 weeks when crusting is beginning to disappear, the pigmentation is starting to go away and the results are becoming visible. Then the last 6 weeks are the 'I love it' phase, because patients acquire a beautiful glow about them.

The skin program can be combined with chemical peels which help to jumpstart the effects of the program. These are carried out every 6 weeks for a course of about 6 months and are very effective in maximising the results of the skin program. I like to use a Blue Peel – but for those who don't want to look like a 'Smurf" I recommend a simple 20% Trichloro-acetic peel. These peels are also great for the back, décolleté, legs, arms and hands combined with the skin program. Peels help to exfoliate the skin and, if a deeper peel is performed, they will damage the dermal layers and cause new collagen formation, reversing the effects of sun-damage.

Another misconception that people can fall prey to is reflected in the incorrect use of bleaching creams: most people tend to apply this only on the pigmented area. Now, bleaching cream works by preventing the action of the enzyme which causes the formation of pigment. If applied on a single spot, the enzyme from the surrounding skin will overwhelm the effects of that bleaching cream. It needs therefore to be evenly applied over the entire face to achieve any results at all.

Exfoliating products freely available on the market can be good unless one overdoes the application and aggravates the skin. While they don't stimulate the build up of collagen, they do get rid of the dead surface cells. However, even using mild exfoliation and avoiding other topical applications such as moisturisers would make a difference to the quality of one's skin. Micro-dermabrasion is an example of a mild exfoliation which if repeated on a weekly basis can improve the texture and pigmentation of the skin.

A lot of women get into the habit of using 'cover up' make-up, such as foundation. A naturally good complexion does not require the use of concealing products. Make up should only be applied in order to accentuate eyelids, eye brows and lips: that is, to accentuate the face, not to cover it up.

Sand-blasting and Cellulite

Micro-dermabrasion (Parisian Peel) or sand blasting can, if used once a week for a period of 6 weeks, help remove surface blemishes. It does not represent a deep correction, but it's a nice non-invasive method and a quick 'lunchtime' treatment. More recently, I found that micro-dermabrasion would remove stretch marks on buttocks and on the abdomen. The treatment smoothes them out and make them less visible so as to almost completely eradicate them. As is the case with facial treatments, one would need to have a session of at least six treatments, once a week for six weeks. Microdermabrasion is not a permanent cure and maintenance treatments are necessary.

Cellulite

Luiz Toledo from Sao Paolo, Brazil developed a device that resembles a pickle fork, with two prongs and a blade between them to divide the attachments of the fibrous bands to the skin (which cause the 'pin-cushion' effect of cellulite). The bands can be parted with the 'pickle fork' and fat injected into the areas to elevate the area.

The Endermologie machine, a combination of suction and pressure, may also improve cellulite. Endermology helps stimulate the blood supply and stretch the fibres that cause indentations and the 'pin cushion' effect in the skin. The patient is given a body garment and the endermologist rolls the device over the appropriate areas, smoothing out irregularities in the process. This treatment is equally good for lymphatic drainage and helps to reduce swelling after liposuction .It has to be noted that the effect is not permanent and regular treatments are needed to maintain it. I recommend two treatments a week for a minimum of 7-10 weeks, and then maintenance once to twice a month.

Botox, Botulinum Toxin Type A.

The other, much-publicised treatment involves the use of Botulinum toxin. Botox is now the most common cosmetic procedure in the world. It works by paralysing the muscles by blocking the release of acetylcholine, a muscle stimulator, from the end of the nerves which in turn causes the muscle to contract. By doing so, it prevents the formation of lines that are themselves a result of muscle contraction.

There are a lot of subtleties and different uses associated with Botox, and constant new applications are found for it.

Primarily, it is used for the horizontal lines on the forehead, the vertical frown lines and the crows' feet. It can also help with the horizontal lines across the bridge of the nose, wrinkly chins, downward slanting angles of the mouth and lines in the neck and it can help raise the eyebrows by applying small injections beneath them. It can even help sweaty palms and sweaty armpits.

The Holy Grail of Plastic Surgery: wrinkly knees, elbows and thighs.

Patients frequently ask me to try out new things. I would consider doing something that hasn't been done before, except perhaps correcting sagging knees and elbows. The surgeon who figures out how to fix wrinkly elbows or wrinkles and fat above the knee cap, will make a fortune. We can take out skin (as we do when we operate on the upper arms, for example) but that leaves scars. Some surgeons claim to have obtained good results using the radiofrequency fat machine, which is akin to a microwave. The results are, however, unpredictable and it is still untried technology.

LASER treatment

Laser resurfacing is a facial procedure that successfully treats deep lines. It is, however, much more invasive than those described above. It can also be used on people who have acne scars, but there is a considerable healing period.

Another option for the deeper lines is the chemical peel. There is a lot of hocus pocus written about these: in the United Kingdom there are a number of 'lay' practitioners with no medical training hyping their 'unique' type of masque or peel. Some of the results I have seen in the magazines have been abysmal.

A Las Vegas surgeon named Gregory Hetter analysed the history of chemical peels and their formulas and concluded in 2002 that the active ingredient was a product called Croton Oil. This was combined in varying concentrations with Phenol, water and soap.

These peels can be performed alone or combined with facial surgery, but there has been no rigorous trials into their effects.

How to look good at short notice ...*without recourse to surgery*
If you had an important event and needed to look especially good
without recovery time, you could do worse than take a leaf out of
the stars' book.

Most actors and actresses would do all they need to do to look
good in the run up to a big event. They would start preparing for
it 2 or 3 weeks beforehand. They would have their lips injected –
perhaps with a combination of Restylane to the edge of the lip and
Perlane to the red part; they would have the naso-labial folds
injected, again with Perlane; and they would go on a good skin
program (if they have 6 weeks to spare); and have a chemical TCA
(Trichloroacetic Acid) or other fruit acid peel two weeks before.
TCA is a fruit acid that peels off the top layer of the skin – it can
also be used to exfoliate at a deeper level. It can go as deep as you
want it to depending on the number of applications. Finally, they
could have a micro-dermabrasion the day before, because it gives
the skin a beautiful glow.

If an average woman with a small budget has the date of her life
and wants to make sure she looks great, she should invest in some
Botox for her upper facial lines and in Restylane and Perlane to
plump up her lips. I would also insist on a course of micro-
dermabrasion: this would not create visible problems on her face,
and she would look good in a short period of time.

At the simplest level, though, a really good hairstyle and hair colour can also do wonders for anyone's looks and confidence.

The tissue fillers

We have a vast range of tissue fillers, but they basically come down to temporary and semi-permanent. There are very few permanent types of filler that I would recommend.

The temporary ones are basically Perlane, Restylane and Juvederm. They can be used to fill depressions, lines and to give fuller lips.

A variation on that concept is New-Fill, or polylactic acid now known as Sculptra in the United States. This is a bit like a fat injection in that it helps to fill the face out in a three-dimensional sense – which is an exciting ability. We can also use New-Fill to build up cheek bones. The result lasts for one to two years but usually requires at least two to three sessions. Another product is Radiesse which is hydroxy-apatite – or bone spheres in a cellulose gel. Radiesse may last several years and is useful again for those nasal labial folds which are the crease which stretches from the edge of the nostril to the angle of the mouth as well as the depression which forms below the angle of the mouth, sometimes know as the 'marionette' lines.

There are newer products such as Isolagen (a culture of fibroblasts from our own skin and Restylane Sub Q which is designed for augmenting cheek bones, but the above are the basic standards. There are many other products available on the market, but the products described above are reliable and safe and give consistent results

With these products we can deal with most problems.

Body

The best way to a great body is the most obvious – regular exercise. However even strenuous daily exercise may not get rid of cellulite. This is where Endermology comes in (*see* above)

In terms of body beautification, I would also mention LASER body hair removal which is very effective. It is better than shaving because it avoids all the associated problems such as infection and pigmentation. It is perfect for smooth legs and the bikini line, or getting rid of the upper lip and facial hair.

Men resort to laser treatment to permanently remove hair on their backs. It is the trend today to have a totally hairless male body and models' chests, shoulders and backs are routinely shaved in compliance with contemporary tastes.

The LASER can only treat hairs in the growth or Anagen phase. Ten per cent of hairs are in the resting or Telogen phase and they will not be affected. Further courses of treatment will be effective when these return to the active phase and grow out. I personally prefer LightSheer Diode Laser, (again, no financial interest) over the pulsed light devices, which I have also used.

Mesotherapy is another fat-shrinking procedure that consists of injecting a product called phosphotidyl choline. Some Mesotherapy treatments are a complete scam, but phosphotidyl choline has been shown to dissolve fat successfully – if only temporarily.

I have tried it on my own 'love handles' and can vouch for its effectiveness. Admittedly it produces a bee-sting feeling and gets hot and swollen and painful. But it only stays that way for about 11 days and then disappears together with the love handles. It is not a totally impressive product, however, in that it is a short term solution. Unfortunately my love handles have returned.

Varicose veins

There is almost nothing better than a great pair of legs – and for women almost nothing worse than having to hide those legs in long pants because of unsightly varicose veins or blemishes. Rather than replacing veins with scars, injection therapy will cure a cosmetic problem with a cosmetic solution. Although it is impossible to 'cure' varicose veins and spider veins, injection therapy – which involves multiple injections over the areas being treated – is probably the most thorough and satisfactory technique for their removal.

The technique was popularised in the 1960s by Professor Fegan in Dublin, who demonstrated that injection plus compression would cause the obliteration of even large varicose veins. Ronald Dee, a General Surgeon in Stamford, Connecticut then published his own technique in 1977 and again in 1999. His technique differed in that he injected the varicose veins every centimetre along their course to ensure complete eradication.. His bandaging technique was unique. Many of the newer techniques employing lasers are just extensions of the 'surgical stripping technique' first described by Babcock in 1907, and essentially unchanged since that date. The stripping technique often destroys the one and only normal vein and a vein that is a valuable resource for heart bypass grafts.

The injection, consisting of the irritant causes the veins to clot and collapse'. They take up to three weeks to disappear completely. The leg is bandaged for a week following treatment, after which the bandage is removed and any blood clots in the veins are extracted with needle punctures to avoid staining of the skin. The leg is then re-bandaged for another two weeks. However, new veins are likely to occur, as no treatment is actually curative. Patients need to return every three months to check for further veins that need injection treatment.

Varicose veins are a problem for both men and women – although in women, they are aggravated by pregnancy. Since men don't get pregnant, they have less common problems with varicose veins. The cause is genetic, and they are not caused by crossing your legs as Nicholas Perricone suggests (this actually increases blood flow in the veins of the leg on top, so cross your legs as much as you like).

Hair restoration for men and for women.
Little-realised is the fact that the incidence of female baldness – or alopecia – increases with age, and in women fifty years and older, some 30% have hair loss, to the extent that they can no longer camouflage it with creative styling. The patterns of baldness vary. Many women have male pattern baldness with recession of the hair line at the top and the temporal areas. Others have a diffuse loss behind the hairline resulting in a widening of the natural part. Fortunately treatment for this can be very effective, and confidence is restored using the patient's own hair as grafts. Hair is removed from the back of the head where it is usually stronger and replaced along the hairline and over the natural parting depending on the pattern of loss. Sometimes only one treatment is required.

Rejuvenating and surgical procedures – the Cutting Edge.
From a surgical point of view, the human face consists of three parts. Beginning at the top and working down, these are: the forehead from the hairline to the eyebrow; the face from the eyebrow to the neck, encompassing the eyelids, cheeks and jaw

line; and finally the neck itself. From an aesthetic viewpoint, however, the face should be viewed as a whole. Picking it apart to do one procedure is like decorating half a room.

Brow lift

The brow is a combination of three elements. One is the hairline, another is the distance between the hairline and the eyebrows, and the third is the level of the eyebrows.

One reason for considering brow surgery is that the brow is too low, or in unusual cases, too high. Another reason is that the patient has prominent frown lines and/or prominent horizontal crease lines at the base of the nose, often combined with horizontal worry lines on the forehead.

The brow lift usually raises the hairline – if somebody has a low hairline with a short distance between the hair and the eyebrows, this would generally be improved by lengthening the forehead and, therefore, they would be a good candidate for a brow lift.

Patients who just have frown lines (without dropping or sagging of the eyebrows) are good candidates for an endoscopic removal of the muscles which cause creasing of the forehead and the horizontal line across the top of the nose. Endoscopic procedures are performed through small incisions, using a telescope whose image is magnified on a TV screen. This way the surgeon can see the nerves and muscles when he operates.

With the endoscopic browlift, staples or stitches are placed in the scalp and taken out in 8-10 days. Endotines are small absorbable hooks which are fixed to the skull using a small drill hole. The brow is then pulled upwards and suspended on the hooks keeping it in position until the brow heals in its new position which takes about 2-3 months. The Endotines devices absorb slowly over a period of a year.

There are two methods of performing a brow lift. One is the endoscopic technique, which uses three small incisions – one in the middle and two about four centimetres on each side – as well as two more incisions in the temple area, one on each side The other technique is called an open brow lift, which involves an incision extending from one ear to the other. This can run straight across the top of the head in a gull wing configuration or extend in a W shape, tracing the edge of the hairline. This hairline cut is especially recommended if the patient's forehead is high, and one therefore wants to avoid elevating the hairline and exaggerating the high forehead.

In the case of an open brow lift, the skin is usually elevated along a natural plane between the covering of the bone (or periosteum) and the fibrous layer of the scalp called the Galea. In the case of an older patient who has lots of lines on the upper forehead, they may benefit from an elevation of the skin in the plane between the skin and the muscle. This will help unfurl and stretch the skin and get a greater smoothing effect in the forehead area. The standard procedure is to perform an incision and elevate the Galea off the periosteum, then remove some of the frown and worry-line muscles from the under layer.

The ideal position of the eyebrow is a slight arch rising from the level of the bony rim of the eye-socket where the brow meets the nose, and then raising *above* the bony rim as it goes outwards towards the ear. The brow is usually at its highest point two thirds of the distance from the nose to its outer point. The brow should finish just above the bony edge of the eye-socket as it tails off. The best eyebrow-waxers recognise this, and taper the eyebrow as it trails towards the outer angle of the eye. They also make the lower edge thinner to give the impression that it is higher. Back in the 1950s and 1960s some women would pluck out their eyebrows entirely and paint them on. Unfortunately eyebrow hair may never regrow – so you must be careful not to get too carried away with the waxer. The same, incidentally, does not apply to pubic or arm-pit hair. Laser hair removal is ideal for pubic and arm-pit hair but is just not precise enough for eyebrows, so the waxers are not going to go out of business yet.

An eyebrow that's low would tend to give the illusion of an excess of skin in the upper lid, or exaggerate an existing problem. It's important not to confuse a patient who comes in asking for an upper eyelid tuck with one who just has a low eyebrow, and primarily needs a brow lift. Most of the time, however, they will need a combination of both.

Equally, with patients who come for an upper eyelid tuck, one should only be cautiously optimistic in terms of the final result. If the brow is low also, the patient should understand that there is room for a limited amount of improvement. Sometimes I would turn down a patient who has very low eyebrows if they only want an upper eyelid tuck because I know they are going to be unhappy with the result. The brow and the eyelids go together as an upper face rejuvenative procedure, often best performed at the same time – in particular the upper eyelids and the forehead area.

Eye-lift or blepharoplasty
In the case of the upper eyelids, generally patients develop excess skin which causes hooding or loss of the visibility of the skin above the eyelashes. This is the area between the eyelashes and the supra-tarsal fold (a nice crease that stretches between the area where women apply mascara and the eye lashes). The crease is usually nine mm above the eyelashes at the level of the pupil and five millimetres above the eyelashes at each angle of the eye. The distance from the supra-tarsal fold to the lower edge of the eyebrow should be no less than one centimeter. Measure yours and see if you comply! Sometimes the supra-tarsal fold may be

elevated when the internal muscle stretches, and this may cause the eyelid itself to droop over the iris and even the pupil. This is a condition called eyelid ptosis or 'sagging', which requires a very specific surgery to repair the muscle that lifts the eyelid. Cosmetic eyelid surgery does not cure this problem so the surgeon must identify the problem and either fix it himself or have a specialist surgeon repair it. The two procedures can be combined.

The stretching and extra folds of this upper eyelid skin prevent the application of mascara and give a rather tired look. Removal of this skin rejuvenates the upper eyelid area. There is frequently a pocket of fat that is removed from the inner angle of the eyelid: it is important not to remove too much fat because this would give a hollowed-out look.

In the case of the lower lid, there are three main problems that occur with age:
One is that the lower border of the eyelid stretches and rounds out, revealing the white below the iris (see page 111). The second is that we develop 'bags' under the eyes. Because these are associated with tiredness, they can give the appearance of permanent exhaustion. The third is redundancy – or excess skin – and the wrinkling of the skin of the lower lid.

There are a number of ways to address each of these issues. For patients who have enlarged fat pads or bags under the eyes, the treatment is to remove the fat. If the patient does not have significant extra skin on the upper lid this can be done through an internal approach.

There are several advantages to this. There is no necessity to create incisions under the eye lashes of the lower lid, recovery tends to be faster, bruising is minimal, and if there is any bleeding it is easily drained through the incision which is left open on the inside of the eye. This operation, which is called 'trans-conjunctival blepharoplasty', does not interfere with the muscle which causes elevation and closing of the lower lid.

So, in addition to removing fat, the other two elements of lower eyelid surgery are as follows: tightening of the angle of the lower lid, which corrects the rounded look and is associated with a more youthful appearance, and addressing the extra skin. Skin marred with fine lines can be addressed simply by re-surfacing the skin with a laser, which would re-tighten the collagen fibres (this does have a downside of possible pigment changes and redness in the early healing period). Alternatively one could use a Croton-Oil peel (*see p. 98*).

A different option is to make an incision in the skin below the eyelashes. The skin is elevated and the extra skin removed. This is a limited technique compared to trans-conjunctival blepharoplasty and laser resurfacing, because with the latter you can avoid injury to the muscle closing the lower eyelid and the risk of drooping of the lower eyelid and it is possible to treat wrinkles extending out in to the cheek and the crow's feet area.

Once again, because the face is a whole and ages as a unit, trying to perform eyelid surgery alone – and in particular lower eye lid surgery on older patients – can be a frustrating procedure. The reason is that as one gets older, the fat in the cheek area drops, leaving us with a visibility of the lower bony rim of the eye-socket, and often what's called a 'tear trough', or depression from the lower eyelid into the cheek. The main problem is that as the cheek drops, so does the eyelid, so trying to pull up an eyelid against the downward pull of the cheek can be a frustrating and sometimes fruitless experience.

The short answer is that when you need a facelift AND an eyelift, don't start with the eyelift. Get both, because the facelift will help the results of the lower eyelift. By performing a facelift and or cheek-lift at the same time as eyelid surgery, one is able to support the lower eyelid and help correct the other deformities of age such as a hollow orbit, achieving better results overall.

The Face-lift

It is a truism that the rich often find the worst surgeons.

I am frequently asked to do repair jobs. Unfortunately not all bad cosmetic surgery – for example a botched face-lift or a rhinoplasty – can be corrected. The motto of a physician is 'primum non nocere' (first, do no harm). When I face such salvage conditions I always wish that these surgeons had done an inadequate job that can be corrected, than performed terrible surgery for which there is no cure.

Even with facelifts that are repairable, a surgeon has to start from scratch and re-do the entire procedure – where the tissues have not been lifted enough, this has to be done properly, and the skin re-draped all over again. A period of at least twelve months has to elapse between two such major procedures.

The more complex the surgical procedure, the longer the recovery period. In order to keep cosmetic surgery enjoyable, if such a term can be used for surgery, recovery time should be reasonable – most people are happy to take 2 weeks out of their schedule, but baulk if faced with a 6-week or even a 6-month recovery time. If the recovery is too traumatic or lengthy, a patient will often be permanently turned off plastic surgery. If they recover fast and have a great result, they will return again and again.

Nothing lasts for ever, though, and none of us will ever be perfect. Ours surgical efforts should be designed to make people look better and stay that way for a reasonable amount of time. Sometimes over-reaching efforts to achieve perfection or a permanent result may do just that, with disastrous consequences. The end-point can be unnatural and mask-like.

Even if a plastic surgeon thinks they know what is appropriate, they need to be mindful of their patients' schedules and imperatives, and take a realistic and pragmatic approach to recovery. One should consider that the ultimate aim is to make people look good – if this look doesn't last a 100 years, then that is fine, for neither do we. A facelift that lasts five years to ten years and has a shorter recovery period is more in keeping with most patient's wishes and lifestyle.

Different people need surgery at different ages. I occasionally see patients now in their fifties who have had facelifts in their twenties, which comes as a reminder that despite our present obsession with the subject, facelifts have been around for quite some time.

Timing

A facelift in one's twenties has obvious limitations in what it can achieve. Nowadays we might suggest a mid-face-lift in the late twenties to early thirty year old as an alternative to a face-lift. The average age for a facelift remains forty-five to fifty-five, even though there is definite trend for starting at an ever younger age.

It is not always a question of timing or chronological age. For example, I recently lifted the faces of a 30-year-old and a 35-year-old. The latter required the rejuvenation effect, but the slightly younger patient simply wanted a more angular face. As I noted earlier, the lines between rejuvenating and corrective surgery are becoming more and more blurred today, because corrective procedures often have the benefit of giving a younger appearance, and vice versa.

Narrow faces can be widened and lifted in the same procedure. Wide faces can be narrowed with fat removal. The tip of the nose can be made smaller and at the same time shortened to make a patient look younger. Sometimes it's just a question of using a procedure that normally makes people look younger to actually make them look different. For example, a facelift in a broader face can give the patient a more East-European look, with higher cheekbones.

Likewise, we can give young patients with a short chin a neck lift, and a better facial line, by using primarily rejuvenating procedures such as chin implants, liposuction of the neck and sometimes a lower face and necklift.

Frequently, when I am doing eyelids, I will tighten the angle of the eye. That's a procedure we use in older patients who have a loss of tone in the lower eyelid, which sags and allows the white of the eye to show below the cornea. Its surgical name is canthoplasty.

Look at the outer angle of your eye where the upper and lower eyelids meet – it should be about 2-3 millimetres higher than the inner angle of the eye. Also, if you look at the horizontal distance between the inner angle and the outer angle, the lower eyelid appears longer and stretched, giving a rounded contour to the outer third of the lower eyelid. Sometimes it's very subtle, sometimes it's more obvious. Generally a youthful eyelid is a tight eyelid, with a nice straight curve from the inner angle to the outer angle. Therefore whenever I do eyelid or facelift surgery I would consider tightening the lower eyelid as well, because it does give a more youthful appearance.

Where a facelift is required for aesthetic, rather than rejuvenating reasons, a patient may want to look different or simply more attractive. They may have a very round face or an obtuse neck that needs tightening. An obtuse neck is one where the chin and neck meet rather like Alfred Hitchcock. A more attractive profile has a defined chin and a near horizontal line beneath it stretching back to a long taught neck. These patients may be in the entertainment industry and, consequently, more demanding about what they want their face to look like.

The most frequently performed surgical procedure – in my practice, anyway – is on the face. Most people assume it would be on the breasts but about twenty-five per-cent of procedures are on the breasts and body.

As we grow older, our noses and earlobes tend to get bigger. Our lips thin and we develop lines that 'bleed' from the red part of the lip into skin around. The jaw line is less defined and we begin to have jowls like Winston Churchill , the brows drop and so do the corners of the eyes and of the mouth. Sometimes the cheeks become hollowed. The whole effect can be rather stern and angry and even pugnacious

As I mentioned above, some plastic surgeons feel they have to do what I refer to as the 'commando facelift'. They would take the whole face apart and put it all back together again in order to create a face that will last for the millennium. I do not believe that that is, practical or desirable. The majority of patients simply want to look better and be able to maintain that look. This can be achieved comparatively easily.

Nevertheless, we have a major dichotomy in plastic surgery right now. We have surgeons on one side who are doing minimal facelift surgery, going back to the techniques that were used on actresses in the 30s, pulling back the skin, putting little stitches here and there and claiming – whether it's true or not – that they get fantastic results. On the other side, we have people who are still doing a major dissection of the face and separating all its many layers, pulling them in different directions. They say they get great results, as well. The obvious question this raises is which approach is best.

What you have to ask yourself is if "A" says they get great results and if "B" says they get great results, how can they both be right? I think the answer is that surgeons who are doing next to nothing are probably getting a very short-lived result. Those who are doing a lot are also getting a very good result that would probably last a very, very long time.

The happy compromise

My philosophy is one of best compromise: that you can get 80% of the result of the more complicated procedure by going half way and getting a quicker recovery. In some people's eyes – both patients and surgeons – it is definitely worth getting the extra 20% and contemplating a longer recovery period, and this is a perfectly justifiable position to take. For me, I don't think that the extra 20% is worth doubling or quadrupling the risks and the recovery time.

In terms of cosmetic surgical intervention, there is no right or wrong choice, rather every surgeon chooses his position in relation to every different patient.

Here is an example to illustrate the above. A patient walked into my office that had seen two plastic surgeons, and I was the third. Each one had told her something different and she was totally confused.

I asked her what the other surgeons had recommended. One had advised her to have a brow lift and a facelift and to have her eyes done; another had told her she just needed to have her eyes done. I told her that she needed to do her eyes and her face.

In this case, these were not really three different opinions, but extensions of possibilities along the same lines – she could do all three, she could do two or she could do just the one. The opinions themselves were not contradictory, rather they all had built-in options. The brow lift I felt was not a particularly strong option, because she was mostly concerned with the eyelids. So, in this instance, I recommended an eyelift combined with a lower facelift.

Ultimately, however, this is a decision a patient should make themselves. The confusion only arises from having to pick a choice from a wide selection. Sometimes it might just be better to get one opinion you trust rather than three you are unsure about. I have a good lawyer, financial adviser, dentist and many other people who form my support team. When I need something from them, I ask their advice and I take it. I don't have the time to shop around anymore. I initially chose them after casting my net wide, but now I have them, I stick with them. I also don't pick my advisers based on false economy: cheap advice and treatment can be worthless.

In terms of a facelift, there are again three elements to a face one might seek to correct.

One is the loss of volume in the cheeks. The second is the drop of the cheek pad which leads to an exagerrated crease between the nose and the angle of the mouth. The third is the jaw line. As the jaw line sags we get jowls forming This is where the cheek falls and meets a doorstop caused by attachments of ligaments along the jaw. The lines that result at the door-stop stretch from the angle of the mouth to the chin – the marionette lines – and these also tend to be accentuated as the jaw line and the cheeks drop. So in summary, the signs of ageing on the face are: hollowing of the cheeks, a flatness of the cheeks as the cheek pad drops; an exaggeration of the lines around the mouth; and often a downturn of the angles of the lips. This occurs with jowling along the jaw line, which loses its sharpness and definition – so that in severe cases it can be difficult to see where the cheek ends and the neck begins and marionette lines from the angle of the lips to jaw. One only has to think of Churchill to visualize all of these changes as he became older until he was the classic English "Bull-Dog".

The other element of face-lifting is tightening the muscles in the facial area. Specifically this consists of tightening the "Superficial Muscular Aponeurotic System" or SMAS for short in the area above the jaw – the angle of the jaw extending up to the cheek bone and to the edge of the orbit. This has several purposes. One is to tighten the jaw line and to help eradicate jowls. Another is to help smooth that nasal/ labial fold which extends from the angle of the nose to the angle of the mouth. The third is to elevate the cheek pads. There are many ways of doing this. The most popular techniques are to either raise this layer off the structures underneath it, mainly the branches of the facial nerve and the major salivary gland, the parotid or to remove a triangle of the SMAS and stitch it up again.

A variation on this theme is to now perform a mid-face lift involving a lift of the cheek fat by elevating it off the cheek bone from an incision in the mouth as well as an incision in the skin of the sideburn and the inner lid and then lifting it and suspending it to the deep ligaments under the scalp.

Having tightened the SMAS, the skin is re-draped. The skin itself is raised up off the muscle for approximately half the distance from the ear to the nose, and is then re-positioned, cutting out the extra skin and trimming it to fit into the cuts around the ear. In order not to create alopecia or baldness above the ear, the skin is either pulled primarily backwards, or it is pulled upwards with a tuck made at the bottom of the sideburn to avoid raising it. In the case of patients with a lot of extra skin the cut is made at the hairline in front of the sideburn, instead of in the scalp area above the ear, so as to avoid giving them a very thin sideburn when the skin is pulled back. When patients have already lost hair in the sideburn area from previous face-lifting, hair transplants can be used to restore the sideburn.

Incisions

Incisions in a facelift can vary. In the temple area, they can extend into the scalp above the ear. The advantages are that the scar will not be visible, a nice smooth re-draping is possible and a pulled aspect of the eyebrow can be created. The downside is that it will thin the width of the hair at the level of the sideburn which can give a 'Facelift look'. The alternative is to perform an incision along the hairline at the sideburn area, which will allow the sideburn to remain untouched – but this has the downside that a thin white line will be visible at the edge of the hairline.

This incision will definitely be preferable in the older patients with extreme skin laxity. Younger patient with less excess skin are more suitable for the scalp incision.

In nearly all of my patients, the incision then invariably extends down on the inner part of the tragus (which is the knobbly bit of cartilage that pokes out in front of the ear canal). The incision is made here so that it's not visible in front of the ear.

The cut then extends around the earlobe and into the area behind, where it ends about where you glasses would end (in the case of a short scar lift). Alternatively it can extend into the scalp area behind the ear. I keep the incision behind the ear high and I make sure that the hair line is matched so that the patient can wear her hair back afterwards.

If the patient has a significant amount of loose skin in the neck, then a standard incision extending into the scalp area behind the ear is recommended. In terms of the closure of the skin, it's very important to close the skin in front of the ear with a stitch which does not leave stitch marks. The stitches are performed under the skin layer and are then absorbed over time without having to be removed. The same applies to the incision behind the ear.

Sometimes I will use a special tissue glue to stick the skin down and reduce the possibility of bleeding. The glue allows the tissues to stick like wallpaper to the underlying tissue. It takes the tension off the repair and reduces the possibility of swelling or bleeding after surgery. Drains may or may not be placed under the skin. If they are, they are usually taken out the next day. The patient generally has a light bandage consisting of a removable elastic strap. Before they go home, they are allowed to have a hair wash by the nurse and I will see them 3-4 days later in my office.

Neck lift

In the neck there are two issues that are important: one is the laxity of the skin itself and the other is the muscle. Frequently the muscle (called the platysma muscle) splits in the middle, leaving two bands or sinews which stretch from the chin down to the base of the neck. If these bands are not repaired and brought back together again, this will lead to an early recurrence of the neck laxity and so, even though you get initially a good result, the improvement will be very short-lived. Sometimes they can be treated also with Botox as a way of postponing surgery.

The way to correct this is to make a cut under the chin and sew the muscles together. Bringing them back together recreates the concavity of the neck. Once this is done, very little else needs to be done to the neck muscle: but the skin itself then has to be elevated from the underlying muscle from the centre point (beneath the chin area), all the way out to under the ears. This is so the skin can re-drape and form a new smoother layer.

Chin Lift

Any attempt to improve the contour of the neck must always include a consideration of a chin implant. As we age the pad of fat in front of the chin drops along with the rest of the face as it loses supporting ligaments and often fat. As it droops, it produces a flattening of the chin and a crease under it. Some people just have poorly developed chins and obtuse necks; both features of ageing as well poor genetics. The solution is to insert a chin implant either through the mouth or through a small incision under the chin, combined with liposuction of any fat under the chin and a neck lift, tightening the muscle and skin in the neck.

Rhinoplasty

There are two age groups who need this type of surgery excluding the broken and the crooked noses which apply to any age. In young adults, the development of the nose can be unattractive and may need to be corrected. A major change like a nose reduction or a chin enlargement is usually far easier for a teenager or a young adult than someone in their 30s or older to withstand psychologically. Body image is much more labile and adaptable in the young. In the older patient, the tip tends to enlarge and drop making the bridge of the nose more prominent and hump-like.

The problems that most people have with their noses fall into two types: one, the most common, pertains to the bridge of the nose, and the other to the tip – which can be too big. Usually we see a combination of the two. There are other permutations still, such as the nostrils being too wide or crooked, or the nose itself being too wide, but the first two are essentially the main reasons for corrective surgery. Corrective surgery is done from the inside usually without any visible cuts on the face – whether to make the tip smaller or narrower, or to make the bridge lower. In addition, the bones of the nose are broken so that the nose will look narrower. That is a good basic operation. The recovery period is about a week.

There are a lot of subtleties to the nose, however. There are patients who don't actually have a big nose, they just have a nose that is unaesthetic and can be improved. It may be a little bit too wide, the bridge may be a little bit too high, the tip may be a little bit too bulbous, etc.

This is the finesse of rhinoplasty – striving to make everything just that little bit cuter.

These, however, are principally the concerns of the Caucasian nose. The other groups that I see are the African or the Asian nose, where the issues are the opposite to those of the Caucasian. Very often the patient will feel that the bridge is too low and needs to be made higher – or more Caucasian. One of the enigmas of plastic surgery is that Europeans want to look more Asian and the Asians flock to their plastic surgeons to be Occidentalised, as it were. A lot of the Asiatic noses are too flat whereas in black noses the nostrils can be very wide and need to be narrowed.

There are surgeons in Hong Kong and Asia in general who specialise in the Asian kind of noses – and there are surgeons in Los Angeles who also specialise in African American noses. Each type presents its own set of problems. Sometimes, a patient will want a change but does not want to lose their ethnic identity, Barbra Streisand for instance.

For 99% of people, the most important facial aspect regarding their nose is their profile. For the other one percent it is the frontal aspect that matters – and they usually tell you which one the moment they walk through the surgery door. They will also tell you what they don't want – most people don't want a ski jump nose, a retroussé type of nose (which is the old fashioned nose), and they don't want flared nostrils, which is also a classic old-fashioned type of nose.

The 'Diamond' nose mentioned in Chapter 2 is a good example of this. Howard P. Diamond did many of the Jewish girls in Manhattan and Long Island, and everybody who was anybody had a Diamond nose – this awful retroussé kind of thing. He would run though High School Graduating classes like a case of Chicken-Pox. To be fair to Dr. Diamond, he did do some fourteen thousand noses during his long career which lasted until the early 1990s. The original look was the way that everyone did them at the time and as he progressed he too changed his outlook and his results. Unfortunately I still see the kind of noses Diamond popularised being done today, although the technique is outdated.

As far as the front-on view is concerned, what patients seek to correct are broad noses, big tips, and tips that droop. People usually want tips that are slightly elevated. It's a sign of youth to have a tip that's up – and a sign of ageing for it to be down.

On profile, women's noses tend to point upwards more than men's. This makes Brad Pitt's nose very feminine and rare for a man of his height: a low bridge, with the tip pointing upward. He looks masculine and sexy no matter what. He has thin hips and a strong chin and jaw line, so he could never be confused with a woman – although I suspect he could do a pretty convincing drag queen act.

The side view is obviously important in terms of how we handle the nose. Importantly, the nose has to be proportionate in relation to the upper lip and the chin. The chin is by far the most important thing to look at when considering correcting the nose. Thus, a lot of people who need nose surgery also need to have their chin done. A small chin makes a big nose look bigger. A small chin with a "beak" line nose gives a bird like profile.

A number of aesthetic proportions have to be observed when performing corrective surgery. The point where the nose meets the forehead, the point where the upper lip meets the base of the nose and the most prominent point of the chin should all form a straight line. If they do not, then one should attempt to bring them into alignment, usually by reducing the nose and making the chin more defined. Often this can be combined with a facelift in an older patient to restore a youthful profile. In the process one can tighten the neck, which is the final aspect of the profile..

While many surgeons measure to achieve precision, I do this by the eye – and know instinctively what is required. I once had a mentor who said that he measured 'scientifically by eye'. He would measure and, then, check visually. For me, the eyes are more accurate than a ruler.

If you make the nose shorter, you can make the upper lip look longer – which may not be a good idea for someone who already has a long lip. With such cases, if you bring the tip up, it would also accentuate the length of the lip and make them look worse. Some people are very astute in appraising their face and many know exactly what is wrong with it. And then again, sometimes they don't.

I had a patient who would have benefited from having her nose narrowed as this would have given the impression of bigger eyes. However, she felt that her face was already wide enough and that such a procedure would make it look even wider. All a surgeon can do is explain the aesthetic considerations – if a patient is not prepared to put the surgeon's judgment to the test, no further influence can or should be exerted. Incidentally, that patient came back and took my advice after her first surgery failed to meet her expectations.

Lips

Men generally prefer bigger lips – as well as bigger breasts – in women. Thin lips and small breasts are simply not attractive to men. This is not set in stone (Julia Stiles and Kirsten Dunst have small breasts and thin lips) but for me there is something very sexy about big lips: Uma Thurman, Liv Tyler and Angelina Jolie are perfect illustrations of this. On the other hand, Melanie Griffiths' swollen lips look awful (though they are now beginning to improve). Antonio Banderas likes his women in the Brazilian mould rather than the London supermodel type such as Kate Moss, and Melanie is doing everything she can to oblige

The best injectable product for boosting the body of the lips is Perlane, or its equivalent. I use Restylane, which is a slightly thinner version of Perlane, to define the margin of the red lip (the red/white margin or vermilion roll). The one drawback to it is that the procedure has to be repeated every 3 to 6 months to maintain the effect.

There are semi-permanent and permanent solutions too. A semi-permanent solution is Alloderm. Alloderm is cadaver (dead) skin from which the antigens (or reactive agents) have been taken out with just the collagen matrix left in order to end up with a sheet of tissue, in other words there are no elements left which can cause adverse reactions. The surgeon then creates a tunnel and threads the sheet in. The whole procedure takes about half an hour to perform, but 4-6 weeks to settle and for the results to be at their best.

I don't like using fat transfer to the lips, because this frequently causes lumps and irregularities. The lip is very unforgiving and if you make a mistake it can be hard to correct. The third alternative is to take a strip of skin and fat without the outer layer of skin, from the lower part of tummy and use this to build up the upper and lower lips. This is probably the best long term solution. It is always best to do both lips since the upper lip which is normally the thinnest, should be smaller than the lower lip. If you just correct the upper lip, there would be a natural imbalance.

There are three ways to deal with the lines above the upper lip. One method is to increase the size of lip and define the margin as explained above. This will correct many of the problems. Another is to inject the vertical lines alone with Restylane. Yet another would be laser resurfacing or a chemical peel.

Mid-Face Lifts

The "mid-face" is the area from the lower edge of eye socket to the level of the upper teeth. In the young, there can be absence of development of the cheek bones so that they appear flat. In these cases I recommend a cheek implant.

When we age or lose weight, the fat over the cheek bones which used to make them prominent, drops and we not only "lose" them but start to get more pronounced lines between the nose and the angle of the mouth and jowls along the jawline. (*see* also the facelift section)

In a patient with minimal laxity of the skin of the face, a good option is to perform a "mid-face" or cheek lift with or without a limited kind of facelift. This cheek lift is done by making an incision in the lower eyelid and separating the cheek from the bone. A second cut is made inside the mouth to free the cheek at its lower aspect and then a third incision is made in the sideburn area so that a stitch or other "device" can be passed from the sideburn area down to the cheek so that the surgeon can lift it up.

The stitch or other device is secured to tissue over the temporalis muscle (the muscle we feel contracting when we chew). This is an excellent option for the mid-thirties group. I was fortunate enough to learn this technique from Dr. Joshua Halpern in Tampa, Florida who is an excellent teacher and a fine physician.

Chins

Chin implants are a fairly frequent procedure. Often they are done in combination with nose surgery or a facelift (see above). One of the problems of ageing is that people get a laxity of the chin pad – and an obtuse angle between the chin and the neck. I call this the Alfred Hitchcock neck because of those wonderful silhouettes that use to appear at the start of his TV serials. Today there are few such people in the public eye: indeed I am at a loss to think of one. This defined angle between the chin and the neck, the mento-labial angle, is associated with youth. As we get older, it becomes obtuse and loses definition. You can tighten it, but a lot of people have aggravating factors such as a very small chin (which tends to produce a convexity of profile). So if we tighten the neck, but the physical distance between the neck and the front of the chin is very short, the only way to correct this is to insert a chin implant.

Usually the implant is a small solid silicone block, which I put in through an incision beneath the chin, right onto the bone. This is a very common procedure. The same can be done for people who need to lend balance to their nose – a common situation as well.

Cheeks

Many patients who need cheek implants need a facelift too, so the most sensible thing to do is to lift their cheeks as part of the facelift operation. (*see* also Mid-Face lifts above)

An alternative procedure that can give definition to the cheeks is to inject filler, such as New-Fill. This is suitable for people who have flatness of the cheeks but do not want surgery. Cheek implants should be used judiciously and never applied to patients who have sunken eyes, as this exacerbates the problem without enhancing their appearance.

A newer product, shortly to be released, called "Restylane SubQ" (a variation on Restylane and Perlane) and a Hyaluronic acid product will also be available for cheeks.

Breasts

There are three types of breast surgery: enlarging, reducing and lifting. They are all straightforward procedures. However if you combine lifting AND enlarging, you combine the complications of two procedures, resulting in a fairly complex type of surgery. This by its nature is a dynamic procedure, one where you push things in one direction and pull them in another, both at the same time.

Breast augmentation is for women who never had breasts to fit their expectations or their proportions or who lost what they had with breast feeding, pregnancy or weight loss.

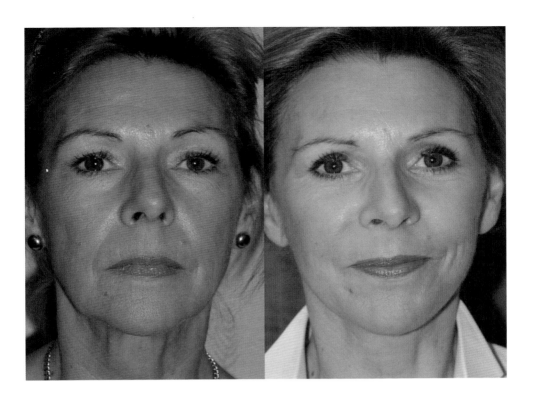

Face-lift, Neck-Lift and Eye-lift, six months after surgery. There were no complications and the patient was very happy with the results.

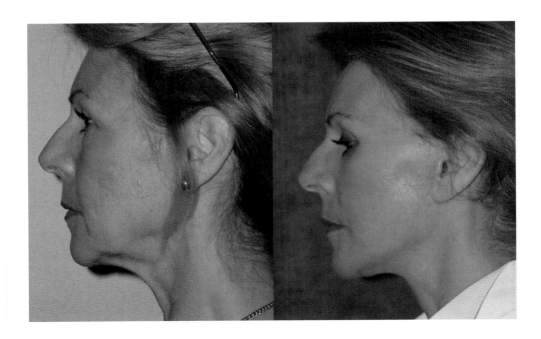

This 36-year-old woman underwent rhinoplasty and the photographs on the right were taken one month after surgery, a classic refined result. There were no complication and I had another satisfied customer.

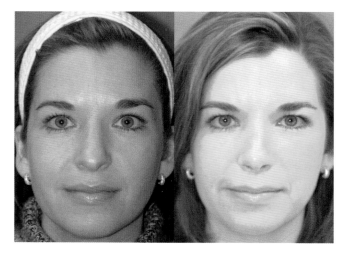

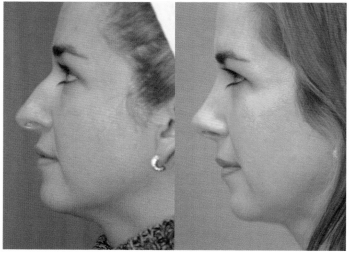

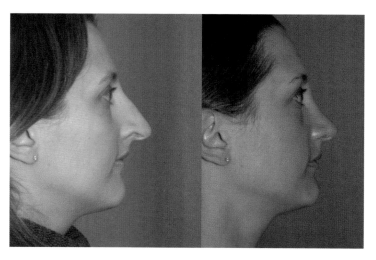

34 year old woman with a very difficult nose... well, for the surgeon. The long tip which had a downward tilt was an aesthetic challenge, which the photographs one year after the operation show that I met.

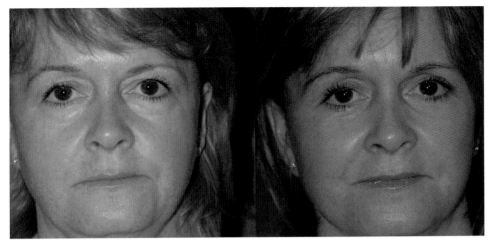

47-year-old after Endoscopic Brow-Lift, Face-Lift with Eye-Lift and Chin Implant with Neck-Lift. There were no post-surgical problems and photographs on the right were taken six months after the operation.

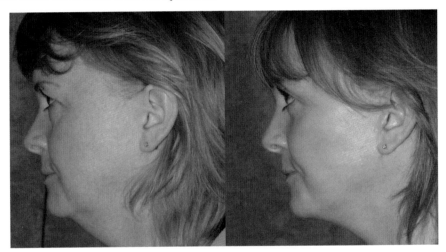

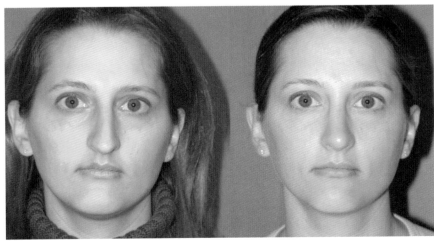

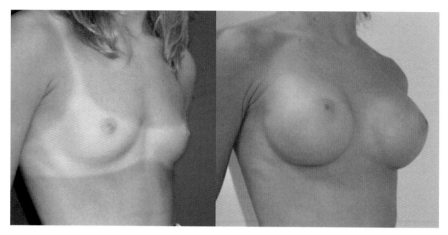

Both young patients underwent breast augmentation, one being more augmented than the other. Both were successful.

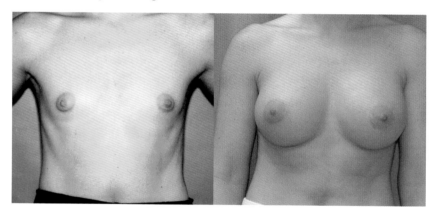

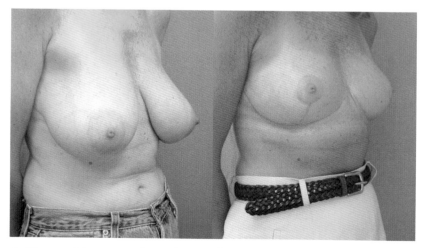

A 43-year-old woman who underwent breast reduction using the standard McKissock technique. The right-hand photograph taken one year after the operation.

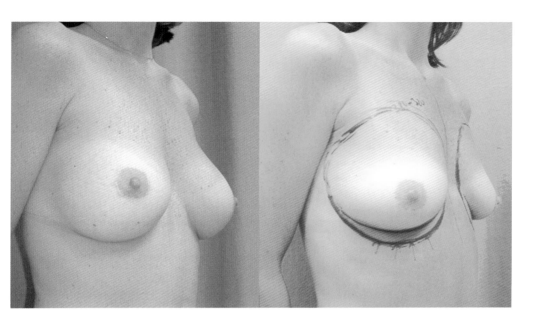

This 33-year-old woman had low profile silicone gel implants under the muscle with areolar incision and peri-areolar lift. The photographs on the right were taken one year after surgery. The operation was successful both aesthetically and medically.

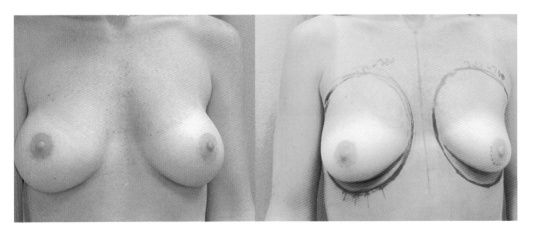

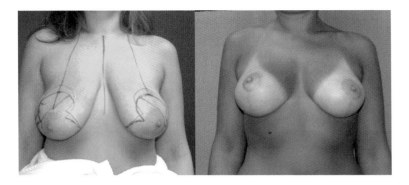

A 31-year-old woman who had a vertical breast reduction. The breasts were reduced and lifted. The photograph on the right was taken six months after the operation.

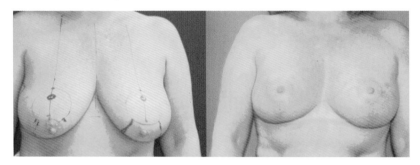

A 45-year-old woman had a similar operation to the above. Again the results were good with little scarring six months after the operation.

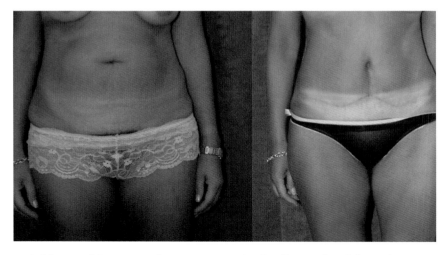

A 34-year-old woman who a tummy-tuck after liposuction followed by a full tummy-tuck with tightening of the muscles, formation of a new belly-button and removal of excess skin.

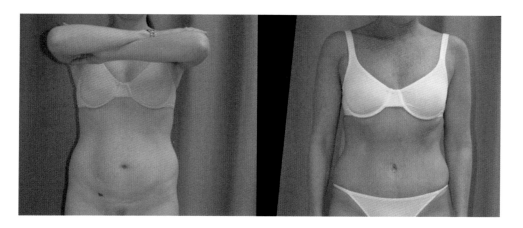

This 33-year-old woman had a tummy-tuck. The first stage [above right], the second [below right]. The operations were separated by three months. The operations were a success and the patient did not put on weight afterwards!

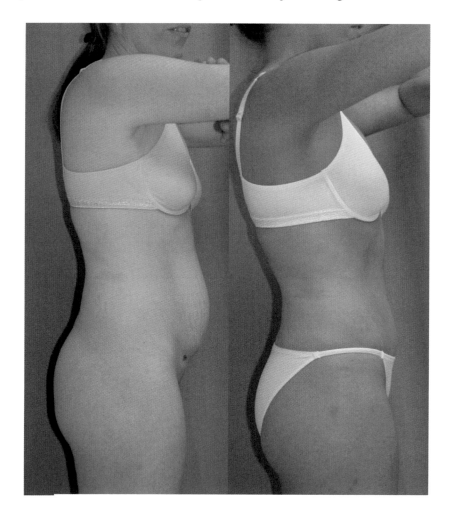

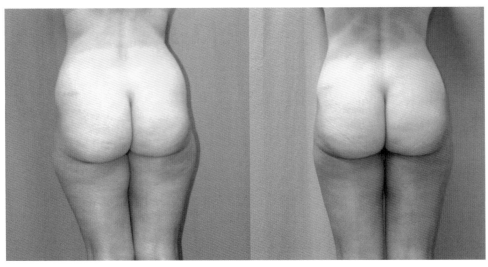

Three-Dimensional Liposculpture of iliac crest (hips), outer thighs, banana rolls and inner thighs, giving the appearance of longer legs. The photographs on the right were taken six months after the operation.

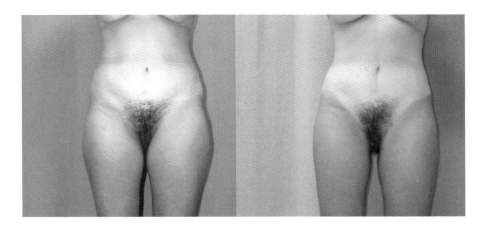

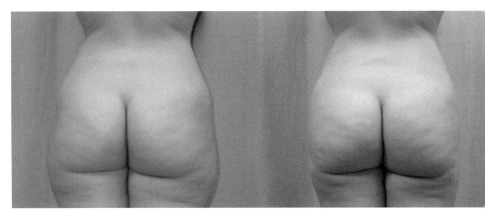

Breast reduction is obviously for women who have large breasts which can begin with adolescence or follow, pregnancy or weight gain. Breast lifting is an integral part of a breast reduction but also applies to those women who have lost support and often volume with breast feeding, pregnancy or weight loss. Some women develop breasts that sag from the beginning without being especially large.

Breast Auto-augmentation (breast lifting using the patient's own breast tissue to create fullness)
A recently developed procedure that gives impressive results in my own hands is the breast 'auto-augmentation' operation. The results of this have been truly remarkable. It is suitable for people who need a lift and more fullness to the breasts, *without* the augmentation aspect of inserting implants. If it is bigger breasts that a patient requires, and then they have to have implants – there is no other way of achieving augmentation. And if they really wanted firmness in the upper breasts then they also require implants.

In a straightforward breast lifting procedure, you can tighten the breast using two techniques. One is to lift the nipple up and to use the vertical scar technique, as popularised by Claude Lassus of Nice, France. The auto-augmentation technique, by contrast, was pioneered in Brazil by Ruth Graff. In this technique the surgeon uses the lower part of the breast as an implant, moving it up, using the breast tissue as filler. The final appearance is that of an implant.

If an implant can be avoided, it should be. Auto-augmentation is not a more complex operation and the complications are much fewer than, say, breast implants combined with a breast lift.

Breast implants

Inserting breast implants is an incredible procedure simply because it works. The current era dates from the sixties. The first implant as we know it today was the invention of Dr. Frank Gerow of Houston. With Dr. Thomas Cronin and Dow Corning, he developed the silicone gel-filled silastic bag which was first reported in 1964. Though there have been modifications, the implants in use today are essentially the same.

However the figures show that every patient who has had it done needs a change of implants ten years later. That said, it is perfect for women who have very small breasts and who feel inadequate or unfeminine. There aren't too many characteristics that distinguish a woman from a man any more – fewer and fewer, in fact. Sometimes it is hard to tell which is which, and it is getting harder. These days even straight guys wear earrings. So, a nice pair of breasts is an asset, not least when buying clothes. The straight guys are still not wearing breast implants.

I favour silicone gel implants. After all the hoopla of the late nineteen eighties and early nineties, the FDA is still waiting for scientific evidence that silicone gel implants cause any long term harm. (The tort lawyers would claim otherwise). However that has not prevented the FDA from keeping them off the market for first time breast augmentation patients. In England and many other countries around the world, silicone gel implants have continued to be available without restrictions.

There are many ways to put an implant in the breast; through an incision under the arm, beneath the breast, through the belly-button, around the areola. My personal preference is an areola incision. In general, I like my implants under the chest muscle because there is less chance of contracture or encapsulation and they don't look like fried eggs on a plate. I prefer smooth implants that are round and I like the high profile type in younger women (before pregnancy, early twenties) and the lower profile in the slightly older group, (after pregnancy, mid-thirties).

I have never really bought into the idea that that rugby ball shaped implants known as tear drop or anatomical implants are more natural or attractive and I usually end up taking them out of unhappy patients. Size is up to the patient, but I suggest bigger because the main complaint after the swelling is down is 'I wish I had gone larger'. If you are going to go through the expense, risk and pain of surgery it is best to opt on the larger side.

Nipple Reduction
(This is a technique that I invented and it is suitable for women whose nipples protrude in an embarrassing fashion. Nipple

augmentation does not seem to be a sought after procedure unless the nipples are inverted and this then requires a correction. We can create nipples, and probably enlarge them by injecting them with Perlane or Radiesse – however, overly large nipples are not within the plastic surgery code. The 'wet T-shirt' look, where symmetrical nipples are standing out nicely is OK, but large nipples are not attractive. One patient who requested a nipple reduction said they were like penises!

Breast Reduction and Breast Lifting

Breast reduction always includes a breast lift. However a breast lift may or may not include a breast reduction depending on the size of the breast.

When I went to "Plastic Surgery School" in Kansas City, Missouri, I learnt the 1972 McKissock (Paul Mckissock, now deceased) technique of breast reduction which involved moving the nipple on the breast tissue below it and tightening the skin with a wide removal in a key-hole shaped pattern that resulted in an anchor-shaped scar. That scar often healed poorly, especially at the inner and outer limits where it was visible. Over time the breast "bottomed-out" so that the nipple was pointing up to the sky and the breast lost its fullness above the level of the nipple.

The technique that I use today owes a lot to Claude Lassus, a Frenchman who with that European flare, refused to believe the dogma of the current teaching and could not accept the awful scars he was putting on to the beautiful breasts of his patients. Instead, he showed us that we could lift the nipple using the tissue above it and then remove the breast tissue below and bring the two sides of the breast together, leaving only a scar around the areola and a vertical scar below it, often completely eliminating the horizontal part of the "anchor".

Over time his breasts did not 'bottom-out' and the patient did not have the unsightly visible scars at the side of the breast and in the cleavage area. There are many other methods but these are the two most common and the McKissock technique is still a reliable technique. For the gigantic breast, the safer technique is to remove the nipple completely as a graft, reduce the breast using either the vertical scar or the anchor technique and then replace the nipple and allow it to acquire a new blood supply.

Tummy Tuck

The American Society of Plastic Surgeons, which compiles yearly statistics on cosmetic surgery, has shown that abdominoplasty (or tummy tuck) is one of the procedures that is dramatically increasing in frequency.

This is because women are becoming less and less tolerant to saggy tummies and stretch marks. The tummy tuck is not a new procedure – it has been around for at least fifty years and the number of patients requesting it has been pretty stable until now. However we have seen an explosion of demand quite recently, pointing to a trend that will eventually see every woman who has had a child consider it – at least once in her lifetime.

Tummy tuck has therefore become a fairly common procedure. There are four aspects to it: one is tightening the muscle when women have a bulgy tummy; another is getting rid of excess skin, fat, or stretch marks; and the third is making a new navel. The fourth is the amount of fat beneath the skin from the bottom of the breasts to the top of the thighs.

The final result depends on what you start with. I have a 38 year old patient who has had a tummy tuck enabling her to wear hipsters with the confidence and appearance of a 20 year old. Not every patient is able to achieve such a remarkable result, however, and should not base their expectations on a surgeon's best-case scenario.

Nevertheless most women would look substantially better after a tummy tuck – a 50-year-old could look like they did at 30 or even 25. Additionally, if a woman is toned and works out at the gym every day, there is no reason why her surgically-enhanced tummy should not look as young as the rest of her.

Women can work out on the muscles in their thighs or their arms, but they can't work out their abdominal muscles once they have been stretched apart, which is why they need this type of surgery. If their abdominal muscles are stretched by childbirth, weight gain or even surgery such as laparoscopic surgery where they inflate large amounts of air into the tummy, they cannot tighten them by exercise alone.

If there is a lot of fat, the final result can be improved tremendously by doing a two-stage procedure. The first stage consists of liposuction of the abdomen. The second stage is the standard abdominoplasty or tummy-tuck in which a cut is made from hip to hip and the skin is lifted up to breasts, cutting around the belly-button. The skin is then pulled down and any excess skin is removed. The vertical rectus muscles of the abdomen are brought back together to create a tight flat tummy. A new hole is cut for the belly-button which is pulled through and made smaller. I like my navels to be vertical. The pubic area and upper thighs are also lifted.

Sometimes a lesser procedure can be performed if the skin is not particularly stretched. There can be removal of skin just in the lower part of the abdomen leaving a short scar about fourteen centimetres long and the muscles can still be tightened.

Arm Lifts, Bingo, Dowager Arms
The procedure of correcting upper arms is called brachioplasty.

This is usually a two-part operation by which you suction out fat and then remove excess skin, leaving the resulting scar on the inside of the arm from the armpit to elbow. The liposuction and the removal of skin are performed at the same time. This, too, is fast becoming a common type of operation as women are no longer prepared to tolerate sagging upper arms ('Old Lady arms', 'Barmaid arms' or 'Bingo Wings').

Buttocks

The buttock is an area that has often been aesthetically neglected. Women have always felt that their bum should be smaller, but attitudes are changing as it becomes fashionable to have a rounded, pert derriere. To achieve the desired appearance, one needs to have a fair amount of spare fat to begin with. This spare fat can be anywhere on the body and is carefully transferred by way of injecting it into the buttocks.

If the bum is sagging, you need to inject fat in the upper buttock, in order to give it a nice curve. This is done carefully by injecting the fat in strips, usually into the muscle where the blood supply is best and the fat most likely to survive

Bums can also get lifted, but this is a big operation. As is the case with all operations, if it is done for the right reasons, the results can be fantastic. The procedure is commonly referred to as the lower body lift. A phenomenal procedure for thin women who have lost a lot of weight in particular, it is often combined with a tummy tuck.

The resulting scar goes all round the waist and can be unsightly, however. One of my patients had a novel solution to this – she tattooed little leaves around the scar. In fact for a time she sported all the attributes of a 35-year-old playgirl – the boy-toy, the Porsche, the fashionable clothes and she was 59-years-old...

Liposuction

Liposuction started as a procedure in the late 70s and early 80s. I was a witness, as a junior trainee in plastic surgery, when it was presented in Hawaii at the American Society of Plastic Surgeons Meeting by the Parisian Yves-Gérard Illouz, in 1982. This really opened the floodgates for a once-sceptical group of plastic surgeons to adopt this technique and start to use it in the United States. There are times in history when we think, foolishly, that we have discovered all we are going to find – and then suddenly a completely new paradigm appears that changes the entire scenery. Consider the horse. There were over a million of them in London at the end of the 19th century: who would have thought that within less than 50 years they would become relegated to ceremonial duties in Whitehall?

The concept of liposuction was rather simple. It meant putting a tube under the skin and sucking out fat using a strong vacuum, close to 1 atm. (standard atmospheric pressure), which liquefies the fat. When it was originally described, a sharp tube was used to cut through the fat without injecting any fluid, which resulted in a lot of bleeding and damaged blood vessels. One also ended up with big spaces under the skin where fluid would collect and slosh around.

It was then discovered that the same procedure could be performed with a blunt tube whilst injecting a lot of fluid containing a minute amount of adrenaline, so as to constrict the blood vessels and reduce blood loss. This helped the tube pass through the fat and also made it easier to suck the fat out.

It was at that point that liposuction was born. It was to become the most common cosmetic procedure, with 60,000 cases a year in the United States alone. Since then the technique central to the procedure has improved a great deal.

Fat occurs in two layers: a superficial layer separated into small pockets, just beneath the skin, and a deeper layer collected together in larger compartments. The original technique involved 'deep' liposuction – the taking out of the deep pocket of fat. Then a surgeon called Marco Gasparotti discovered that superficial liposuction was also important. This meant suctioning under the skin to help contour the overlying skin. This was tremendously important conceptually, as well as a step forward in the sophistication of technique. Liposuction was no longer just fat removal but fat *sculpting*. It had to take an Italian with the blood of a Bernini to think of this!

Marco Gasparotti and I co-wrote a paper explaining the concept of shaping a body through sculpting, using this method. called Three-Dimensional Liposculpture. I was fortunate enough to train with Marco in Rome, and I think that he would agree with me if I said that he does his body-sculpting like a rhinoplasty.

Since then there have been further advances. For example, at the beginning, the only way to get at the fat was with a cannula, moving it back and forth with the strength of your arms – a technique that is physically very strenuous. We now have various devices that replace such exertion. There exists a device called Power Assisted Lipoplasty (or PAL) which is an electrically powered handle that drives the cannula or suction tube back and forth at 4000 times a minute. This makes the passage of the tube easier and also allows us to take fat out in a more even fashion, with less trauma and less bruising.

There are other methods of taking fat out. There is ultrasound, which transmits an ultrasonic wave that liquefies fat, but I have never been a great fan of that – I just don't feel that I have the visual feedback that I need to sculpt. The ultrasound liquefies the fat in a rather gross fashion like melting jelly. It then has to be removed by suction. For me Lipo-sculpture is more akin to eating cheesecake with a spoon, shaving off flakes as you devour it. A new liposuction device proposes to drive in fluid under pressure as you suction out the fat so that no injection of fluid is required beforehand. This could be another Eureka moment.

THE PRICE OF BEAUTY

The best things in life are **not** free

Myth and Reality Shows. Life imitates TV

There are at the moment more than a couple of 'reality' TV shows in the US, *Extreme Makeover*, *The Swan* (soon to be shown in the UK), *Dr. 90210* (the Zip code for Beverley Hills) that go a long way towards popularising plastic surgery and to demonstrating what it can achieve. As we go to press, Channel 5 is following suit over here, with its sensationalist *Plastic Surgery Live.*

Extreme Makeover is an HBC program that encourages people to send in pictures or videos of themselves explaining why they think they are good candidates for a total makeover. The concept of the program is a good one, in that it allows people, blighted by real or imagined imperfections. to step out and have them corrected for free. In combination with surgery, the show offers them advice on diet, fitness programs, clothes, make-up, grooming... just like I do.

The program makes sure that all the patients are evaluated by a psychologist and a psychiatrist. Then they are all evaluated by plastic surgeons certified by the American Board of Plastic Surgery, who are also members of the American Society of Plastic Surgeons (ASPS). Patients have to be deemed acceptable to the plastic surgeon in order to have surgery – this is a bit like winning a lottery ticket. Strangely the ASPS specifically proscribes its surgeons from participating in a lottery-style selection process. Some were ostracised and subsequently resigned from the ASPS in disgust – whilst others were allowed to fly beneath the radar. But the ultimate benefit is that the surgeons chosen were suitably qualified to perform the surgery.

The Swan is a similar concept with a slightly different angle. The most significant gimmick is that patients take part in a beauty pageant after completing their 3 months of surgery, recuperation and grooming. The program draws its surgeons from specialties other than Plastic Surgery. Of course, the end results depend vastly on what potential the patient had to start with. It's the hand with which you are dealt that determines the outcome of the game.

Some have said that shows like *Extreme Makeover* are a ticking time-bomb for an Extreme Death. Certainly there is a flipside to such TV programs, and I would say that they create some dangerous misconceptions. One is that a great deal of surgery can be performed within several hours without any danger of increased complications. One of the most common reasons for significant complications in plastic surgery today is combining too many surgeries at the same time. This at a time when we see a lot of serious complications or even deaths in the United States as a result of cosmetic surgery.

Is it 'extreme' lack of judgment to perform an abdominoplasty, breast lift and a facelift at the same time? I think so. Ultimately the patient takes longer to recover and comes out of the experience (assuming they survive) with the sworn intention never to repeat it. It would be perfectly fine to do these procedures separated by a day or two, and that is the way they should be done. Sadly it just would not have the same impact on TV viewers. In real life patients undergo extreme makeovers– they just happen a bit at a time.

Another misconception these shows create relates to the cost of cosmetic surgery. Most people have absolutely no concept of what a complete makeover would cost. The man in the street doesn't have the resources for such extensive surgery, which would cost a minimum of £120,000. The average dental re-fit alone is the cost of a Porsche.

Frequently, in the aftermath of a TV show such as *The Swan*, people will go to a plastic surgeon's office, influenced by the transformation they have witnessed on television. They demand a makeover style procedure, expecting the cost to be in five figures.

The reality of cosmetic surgery is different – it is very expensive. These TV shows can distort people's expectations without educating them about the real cost and dangers involved. Practically speaking, extreme makeovers are beyond the realm of most people's financial ability.

My advice is: don't make your appointment at the plastic surgeon's surgery (or office, as we call it in the States) till you've cashed in your pension fund! And don't vent your anger on him when he hands you the estimate of the cost. Think about cosmetic surgery like buying a car, except it will last ten years instead of three to five.

Surgeon's fees

A curious phenomenon I have seen in patients is that as they request more and more procedures they expect the fee to decrease with each additional item!

When we talk about cosmetic surgery fees, it is important to separate the surgeon's fees from the costs of anaesthesia and hospitalisation.

Hospital and anaesthesia costs change – they can range from £2000 to £3000 or even more, combined. Anaesthesia costs are from as little as £300 for a breasts augmentation to as much as £1200 to £1500 for a facelift with a browlift and/or chin implant.

This is because one takes an hour and a half, and the other may take 6-8 hours.

The hospital fee for a breast augmentation would be about £1450 for a one-night stay. If a patient is going to have a brow, facelift and eye-lift surgery the fee would be £2400. Obviously, the more procedures a patient has, the more it costs, but there is a definite saving to the patient by combining several procedures at the same time. If they chose to have their eyes done first, then the face and later the nose, it would cost them three times as much in hospital fees. The final fee really depends on the hospital and what the hospital feels the market can bear at any one particular time. The same applies to fees set by the anaesthetist. And remember all fees are estimates until you book the surgery and, yes, unfortunately fees go up over time, so if you decide to postpone surgery for several years, expect to pay more when you return.

The surgeon's fee is fixed according to what the surgeon feels he is worth. When I put a fee on a procedure, it doesn't mean that a patient couldn't pay a lot more – or a lot less. Every surgeon has a fee based on what he can command.

If a surgeon can command a certain fee for a facelift and patients are willing to pay it in enough quantities – such that he doesn't have available space to operate on anybody else for the next 3 months – then obviously there is no reason for that surgeon to reduce his fee.

On the other hand, if someone charges the same and has no patients on his schedule, he would clearly have to drop his fee.

If a patient informs me that they can get the same procedure done next door for a thousand pounds less, my answer is always, 'Then, by all means, that's clearly the person you should see, because if these are your criteria, I am not the surgeon for you.' Hiring a surgeon is not like buying a car. You are buying expertise, trust and a very individual experience. If a patient feels that they would be getting the exact same quality of advice and expertise wherever they go, they would not be coming to me.

Some surgeons feel that they prefer to operate on a larger number of patients and spend a shorter time on each, charging a smaller fee to do so. For my part, I've never liked mass-produced medicine. I've always enjoyed patients – talking to them, learning about them, getting to know them. Some of my patients have become friends or business associates. I see them as patients but frequently I just spend time chatting to them because I enjoy talking to people. One couldn't do that if one had to see ten people an hour.

Patients for their part appreciate being listened to, without being rushed or being treated as crackpots. They usually can tell you more about their aesthetic problems and what they need frequently from a very accurate viewpoint, if you are prepared to listen. On the other hand, that is no excuse to prattle on about every

THE PRICE OF BEAUTY

irrelevancy because then the surgeon is forced to ask direct questions, such as 'why are you here?'

I generally try to see the reasonable side of anybody, even if my first impressions may sometimes be negative. I would listen and try to understand and get an angle from the patient's point of view, to understand what drives them. I am not always successful – there are people that I detest and who doubtless feel the same about me, and that's always going to happen – but in general that's my philosophy and my approach to surgery.

It is fair to say that I am never going to be a cut-price plastic surgeon, but nor am I trying to be the most expensive one. From the very first day I began in practice I have set my fees at the higher end and I don't think that it has ever affected the number of patients I have seen. Surgeons who set their fees lower may give a subliminal message which says either 'I am not very good at this' or 'this is my second job, so anything in the can is welcome'.

Cosmetic surgery is my 'day' job. I don't have a full time consultancy in the NHS. If I did it would materially affect my ability to give my best efforts to my cosmetic patients. In the US, I gave up many aspects of my practice of reconstructive and hand surgery so that I could devote the best hours of the day to cosmetic surgery. Any cosmetic surgeon should do the same. It is not a part-time job. Nor should it be a night-time job.

Some cosmetic surgeons restrict their practice to an even greater degree: Howard Diamond, Gustave Aufricht and Jacques Joseph, devoted themselves to noses; Marco Gasparotti, in Rome specialises in the 'Three-Dimensional Liposculpture' technique; Dan Baker in New York does mainly facelifts; Alfonso Barrera in Houston, Texas, specialises in hair transplantation and so on. My practice is 75% facial plastic surgery including noses, facelifts, brow lifts and eyelifts. The balance is made up by breast surgery and body contouring, such as tummy-tucks and liposuction.

A price guide

If you were like me and tend to read books from the end back to the start, you would be reading this first. Having explained the principles behind charging, here is a menu of surgeon fees for the majority of procedures described in this chapter. Please note that except where specified, these are surgeon fees *only*, not the total cost of the procedure. I have given a range because each case is unique and presents its own individual problems.

Facial procedures:

Rhinoplasty: £4000 - £6000

Eyelids: £3000 -£4000

Facelift: £6000 - £8000

Browlift: £3000 plus Endotine implants (see above) £350

A facelift, browlift and eyelift: £10000

Otoplasty (pinning back the ears): £4000

Liposuction under the neck: £1500

Chin implant: £1500

Cheek implants: £3000

Mid-Face Lift: £3000 plus Co-Apt implants (see above) £350

Non-surgical treatments:

Remember that you are not paying for the syringe but the injector. There is a clip in a Danny Kaye movie where he plays a hairdresser and creates some incredible hair do on a woman and tops it off with a little ribbon. The woman's comment when she hears the price is 'That is a lot of money for a ribbon!'

Kaye's response is 'Madame, the ribbon is free.'

Perlane / Restylane: £375 a syringe

(A patient usually needs 1-2 syringes of each, Perlane and Restylane)

Botox: £250 per area, Forehead, Crow's feet, Glabella frown lines etc.

(Botox is usually needed in 1-3 areas)

Radiance: £1200 per syringe (more because this is a semi-permanent solution)

New-Fill: usually £600 to £1200 per treatment (and requires 2 to 3 treatments to get the final result). This is now known as Sculptra in the United States and marketed by Dermik and a division of

Aventis Pharmaceuticals.

Alloderm to the lips: usually £2000 (plus the product which costs an additional £400)

Dermal grafts to the lips: usually £2000

Other surgery:

Breast enlargement: £3500

Breast reduction: £6000

Breast auto-augmentation: £5000 -£6000

A breast lift of any kind, with or without an implant: £5000 (in addition to the cost of implants which are approximately £500 to £800 for the pair)

A nipple reduction is £1500 – £2000.

Lipoplasty /liposuction: about £2000 per major area such as the abdomen, the outer thighs, the hips (described as the iliac crests) and the flanks combined (the area under the bra-strap). Minor areas such as the inner thighs and knees are £1000 a pop.

Combined procedures are priced as follows: Thighs, iliac crests and flanks approximately £3000 to £4000, Abdomen alone £2000 to £3000. Liposuction, therefore, can cost between £2000- £6000 and can be combined with fat injections to the buttocks, (in which case I would not necessarily charge an additional fee)

Because of the subjectivity of liposuction and the fact that unfortunately not everybody maintains or loses weight after it, I don't offer to perform further liposuction at no fee. From my viewpoint there is always a fee to remove fat. Secondary surgery is however usually half the cost of the original.

Brachioplasty (removing the skin from sagging (Bingo) arms): £5000 –6000

This is quite a lengthy procedure and takes about 2 hours for each arm

Tummy-Tuck: £7000-8000.

Lower body lifts are about £12,000 – thigh lifts alone are about £6000 and I charge a lot because they are tedious to do.

Varicose veins: £4000-5000 per leg.

This is a procedure based on injection therapy. Again my fees are higher than many because I treat a whole leg at one time and not in multiple treatments – which frequently end up costing more and being ultimately less effective, like polishing a car one door at a time. My original fee includes unlimited injections and office visits for the following twelve months.

LASER hair removal, because it requires multiple treatments, can be quite expensive. It starts at £500 but can end up costing £2000+. LASER skin re-surfacing for deep lines is about £4000 for the entire face or £1000 for the area just around the mouth.

Additionally, there is a whole new field of gynaecological cosmetic surgery. I work closely with a gynaecologist in the United States who has a Vaginal Rejuvenation Institute. He performs such procedures as labioplasty, tightening of the vagina, augmenting the G-spot and reconstruction of the hymen. The cost of a vaginal rejuvenation procedure is £3000-£8000 and many English people are beginning to travel to the USA for this type of surgery. For more information on this please contact my office.

If these prices seem out of whack, it is worth noting that celebrities tend to get charged more – by most surgeons, whether the surgeons admit it or not. This is for two reasons: firstly, they can afford it, and secondly many of them require a lot more hand-holding. Sometimes though, a celebrity will be charged next to nothing if the surgeon can broadcast the fact that he did it, as was the case with Tom Loeb, M.D. and Linda Tripp of Monica Lewinsky and Bill Clinton fame.

To balance the books, students and nurses slide by at a discount. The other category are known as 'wactresses'. This a common type in New York City, referring to aspiring actresses or actors in servile jobs as waiters or waitresses, but who may one day be famous (and they also have a lot of similar friends!). For this reason they usually get a healthy discount. Tom Cruise, for example, worked as a janitor until he got his first break.

Plastic Surgeons still do spend a proportion of their time rushing off to Eastern Europe or South America to do charity surgery on children and adults on a pro bono basis.

I set up a charitable arm of 'Americares' an American Charity, entitled 'Doctors for all People' and in 1989 found myself in the middle of the earthquake disaster in Yerevan, Armenia. I still get letters of thanks and gratitude from those patients.

In 1993 and 1995 I organised two missions to Rijeka in Croatia, under the auspices of UNESCO to operate on war injuries and other plastic reconstructive problems. Working in conjunction with Mario Zambelli, the local and very talented Chief of Plastic Surgery, we transplanted a toe onto a young man's hand who had lost his thumb in a bomb blast; and we were the first surgeons to perform breast reconstruction using an abdominal muscle flap helping many women who had desperate deformities after mastectomy for breast cancer.

Length of Surgery:

Some surgeons are faster than others. Speed is neither an indicator of excellence nor vice versa. Each of the described surgical procedures usually requires a night stay in hospital in the United Kingdom. In the United States most procedures are performed in my own private surgical centre under sedation and the patient often goes home or to a local hotel afterwards. Recovery in all cases means return to work or social schedule.

Rhinoplasty: an hour and a half (recovery one week).

Face lift: three and a half hours (recovery: two weeks).

Mid- Face Lift: one to two hours (recovery: 2 weeks).

Brow-Lift: one hour (recovery: one week).

Eyelids: one hour (recovery: one week).

Chin: thirty minutes (recovery: one week).

Otoplasty: one to two hours (recovery: one week).

Breast enlargement: one hour. Breast reduction or a lift: three to four hours (both recovery: one week).

Tummy tuck: three and a half hours (recovery: two to three weeks).

Liposuction: anywhere between one and three hours (recovery: one week).
Body lift: four to five hours (recovery: two to four weeks).

Fat injections in the buttocks do not require a hospital stay.

Recovery time for the majority of operations such as these will be approximately one to two weeks, and people can look more or less normal after that period of time.

Back to the future
We are always quick to claim to be the first and yet it is surprising how many of our new techniques were described decades or centuries ago. So anything I claim to be new here may well be old-hat and I apologise in advance to my predecessors if I omitted to give them due credit.

In my opinion the future trends of cosmetic plastic surgery will focus on less invasive surgery – in fact on less surgery altogether.

There are now barbed threads designed to lift the face and even the buttocks. No-one is really sure as to how effective they will be long term. Hyaluronic acid-based products, or other kinds of natural substances, may gradually replace breast and facial implants. Soon we may be able to inject breasts with Macrolane (a form of Hyaluronic acid), when augmentation is desired.

Poly-lactic acid is already being used to increase the volume of the face in older patients, and other new applications will be developed for this product. This trend of using bio-compatible tissue fillers to replace lost volume in older faces, or to build up volume and correct the collapse of the face, will continue.

Using our own tissue by growing it in the lab, for example Fibroblasts grown in tissue culture from our own cells, to re-inject and rejuvenate the skin – another innovation that will be increasing in popularity.

All of the 'short-scar' techniques will be used increasingly. The traditional facelift, for example, has a scar that goes round the ear and into the scalp behind the ear. By using a short scar technique, this scar can stop behind the ear without the final effect being in any way compromised – quite the contrary, in fact.

This is a significant advance in terms of procedures, even if it hasn't been adopted by all surgeons. The standard facelift incisions are still used to great effect on the patient with a very slack neck and a lot of extra skin. Sometimes the neck only is treated, resulting in a scar which starts just at the earlobe and snakes around behind the ear and into the scalp.

As in all disciplines, some people are slow to embrace new developments, and I occasionally see results of the old-fashioned style of rhinoplasty which mainstream surgeons abandoned 25 years ago. Short-scar facelifts and short-scar breast lifts are here to stay, and we will see much more aesthetic and effective results because of this. Vaginal rejuvenation, buttock augmentation, body-sculpting and body-lifting are all procedures that will continue to improve. Anal rejuvenation surgery for the gay community is probably next on the agenda. Doubtless I will have been long retired before I am called upon to perform such life-enhancing operations.

More generally, as time goes on, people will simply be more demanding about their bodies. Unfortunately, there are those of us who are never going to look like a supermodel no matter what we do. If one is built like a wine barrel, all one could possibly hope for is to look like a *thin* wine barrel.

The Russians have developed a method of stretching the bones in order to add height, but this is such a lengthy, painful and tedious operation to perform that most people would not consider it – unless they were vertically-challenged to the extreme.

In the last couple of years, there has been a flood of conflicting information on human growth hormone (HGH) and its restorative powers.

HGH will not yet replace cosmetic surgery to become the magic solution of the future, not least because nobody knows what the long term effects of it are. The few patients I have had who have been on HGH acquire a distinct and peculiar look after a while. Certainly, I would neither prescribe this, nor use it myself. The science is still not convincing that HGH is the elixir of youth.

LIFESTYLE

Do I have to go to the gym every day?

You might wonder, why come to a plastic surgeon for tips on health and nutrition, on lifestyle, exercise or fashion? You may wish to employ your own 'Lifestyle guru'. But the simple fact is that many people come to my surgery expecting to look better, and willing to pay through the nose for it, when they are forgetting some of the basics of how to dress, eat and look after themselves. There is no point wasting energy on a physical specimen that will go to pot anyway. So here is my guide to living a better life for your own body – and first, a checklist of what to get straight before you make the leap into my office.

Before you resort to surgery

Or what you can do before you get there to improve the way you look.

Read *What Not To Wear* by Trinny Woodall & Susannah Constantine, Weidenfeld Nicolson (no, I don't have an interest).

Lifestyle and diet

No sun-tanning; artificial tans only.

No smoking.

One glass of wine with dinner, maximum.

A good night's sleep (invest in a great bed, and the most expensive sheets, duvet and pillows you can find, makes for great sex. Oh, and Harvey Nichols for bed linen).

A regular exercise routine.

A diet low in high-glycaemic carbohydrates, rich in ocean-caught fish and olive oil.

The use of vitamins, minerals and nutritional or diet supplements

A healthy set of teeth.

A good-looking set of teeth aligned and filed down (see a cosmetic dentist and an orthodontist).

Hair: for women

Hair length:

a. long neck = shoulder length.

b. Short neck = earlobe length.

Hair colour:

a. pale skin = lighter hair.

b. darker skin = darker hair (avoid contrasts).

Hairstyle:

a. wide cheekbones = thinner, longer cut.

b. low cheekbones = fuller, shorter cut (both depend also on neck length – *see* above).

Hair and ears:

Get a good expensive hair cut.

Avoid long straggly hair (only the very young can have long hair and even then often not).

Your ears were not designed as hooks that stick out to keep the hair off your face.

If you have small ears and earlobes, show them off, enhance with delicate earrings.

If you have big ears and big earlobes, or bat ears: don't draw attention to them.

The alternative is to hide them with a longer cut.

Forehead:

High forehead with lines: brush hair forward or centre-part

Do not pull back, but avoid heavy fringes.

Beauty and unwanted hair in odd places:

Facial hair is unacceptable in women, laser it off or pluck it.

Wax your eyebrows and body hair: at the most a landing strip (don't ever find yourself asking, should I have shaved?)

LASER hair removal, waxing or depilatories. LASER hair removal is the best if you are a good candidate for it: pale skin, dark hair.

Your underarms and the skin of your thigh below your panty line should always be shaved or LASER'd. Even men now are shaving their body hair.

Grooming: Yanks v Brits

While cosmetic surgery is by no means available to everyone, it should not become the visible class divide of the future. We live in an affluent society and people have disposable income to choose how to spend. Just as some people choose to spend it on a holiday or on a car, others would go for plastic surgery.

Although you would never be able to afford cosmetic surgery on benefits, people of all backgrounds do choose to spend money on surgical enhancements. If a social divide does exist, it is certainly not as wide as one might assume. Rather, there is a cultural divide in terms of grooming. To illustrate this, one only need to compare attitudes in England to those in North America.

A standard joke in the States is that the English can only afford expensive petrol because they scrimp on personal grooming (although maybe Americans need that cheap fuel because they spend so much on their appearance!).

English politicians – both men and women – are remarkable for their lack of grooming. In fact generally in this country those in the public eye probably do not devote enough time or resources to looking their best. The fashion industry would be the obvious exception to this, while many in TV, for example, look positively dowdy. Stephen Fry is a good example. His nose is incredibly crooked, yet one could make an allowance for it because the nose has become part of his personality as an actor. This does not excuse the fact that he is overweight, though – especially since he has taken on the role of Sherlock Holmes in a forthcoming ITV series. Holmes is described as a lean man in the books – a fact Fry at least acknowledged when he said, 'There's no mention at all in Conan Doyle of Holmes being a wobbly lard-arse, so I'm going to have to get tuned-up in some horrible way.' This is typical of the English aversion to exercise and grooming.

Looking at some of the English TV presenters, again Eamonn Holmes is on the heavy side. His female counterpart Fiona Phillips has a beaky nose and crows' feet that ought to be fixed. I guess this is just the expatriate Brit in me speaking, in that I no longer find the crooked toothy smile and horsey profile attractive! Compared to soap actors in the States, English actors fail miserably in the grooming stakes – and this is even without taking into account surgical enhancements.

There are of course exceptions, thank God. I have already mentioned Kristin Scott-Thomas, Diana Rigg and Julie Andrews as some of those who have maintained their looks through well-judged surgery. Jemima Goldsmith is obviously going to keep herself in better shape than her mother. On the other hand, there are those who have succeeded in Hollywood with visual deformities. Joaquin Phoenix has made a spectacular career with a repaired cleft lip which is quite visible. Stacey Ketch did the same until his drugs and drinking got in the way. Chiwetel Ejiofor, the lead in *Dirty Pretty Things*, has multiple scars on his forehead from a childhood car accident but has had a succesful acting career.

Male actors have a peculiar grooming affectation that seems to go with the profession – they tend to dress all in black from head to toe. Yet there is nothing especially stylish about this – rather than enhancing one's looks, the main effect of black clothing is to emphasise a man's dandruff.

The average English male looks like he got dressed and then had a ten minute nap before he left the house for work. However, the quintessential Bond type is still perfectly groomed (with the square, dimpled chin and – curiously for an Englishman – black hair).

General grooming guidelines

When women walk into a plastic surgeon's office and ask for advice, this is because they are unhappy with their looks. They ask what can be done to improve their appearance and typically, if there is a list of five items, chances are that at least two surgeons would recommend the same course of action. However, few women walk in and says 'make me more beautiful'. Rather, they will mention a well-known person's best feature and request the same. As a plastic surgeon I frequently ask women to observe a few general grooming rules: It is a mistake, I feel, for older women to wear ultra short skirts even if they have good legs. Tina Turner is a case in point. She has great legs and can get away with it, but then she has a thick trunk. Many women have great legs in older age and can still show a bit of thigh, but I feel that it would be to their advantage to cultivate a more sophisticated look rather than an overtly sexy one. It is a mistake to try and look like a siren past a certain age… whatever age that may be!

If a woman of 50 tries to look like someone in their twenties, she looks exactly like a 50-year-old trying to look like a 20-year-old. However, if she aims to look 30-40, then she can do so fairly effortlessly – and the result is far sexier and more aesthetically pleasing. Indeed, I know 50-year-olds these days who have great bodies. They can compete with 30-year-olds and they would probably compete even better if they have taken care of themselves and had the help of plastic surgery.

Another recommendation is that the older we get, the shorter our hair should be. This is for several reasons: because it makes us look younger, because we need to change our style every so often during our lives (but reach a point where we would rather keep it manageable), and also because hair doesn't have the same consistency. It won't fall the same way it did when we were younger.

Hair becomes a big issue for men as they grow older. Unlike with women, grey hair looks good on men – and when they dye it they just look silly. Having said that, President Reagan (who had a great head of hair for his age) did his so professionally that it always looked great.

Long hair in a man also looks silly, as do pony tails, and this becomes especially true with age. Still, shaved heads and very short hairstyles are also not attractive in men – even if you are a Brad Pitt fan. A short haircut is fine, but not a cropped cut.

It is worth noting that – ageism in the workplace notwithstanding – our perceptions of how old means *old* are also changing, to reflect advances in rejuvenation procedures and increased lifespan in general.

In my opinion, piercing of any kind is extremely unattractive except in the ears of women. Piercing in the nose is only acceptable in an Indian or African woman, because this is culturally appropriate. In a white person, piercing in the nose, tongue or anywhere else is aesthetically offensive – and the same goes for tattoos. They stay forever but never look good. It's like reading yesterday's newspaper, every day.

For both men and women, weight is THE issue of the century.
Slim is in, Fat doesn't fit. And yet we abhor anorexia. The fashionable clothes that are made today don't fit fat people – but while everyone wants to be thin, not everybody can be. Neither

should they be – just because we see an ideal, it doesn't mean that we *have* to look like that ideal. There are people who are happy with the way they are, and if this is the case, the only reasons to change it would be medical. No plastic surgeon would tell a patient to change themselves if they are comfortable with the way they look. However, being overweight poses significant health risks: so fashion aside, everyone has a reason to be at least trim. The best test to see if you have any extra fat, is to strip naked and jump up and down in front of the mirror. If you can see the lag between you and your fat reaching the end point of each trajectory, then you need to lose weight.

The only way to permanently lose weight is to adopt a healthy lifestyle. In the next section, I will devote a few pages to exploring what this means from a medical standpoint.

Exercise and health supplements, diet, lifestyle

Most of us equate looking good with feeling sexually attractive. Looking good and being fit both require a great deal of effort. Working out at the gym, for example, is something a lot of us elect not to do.

For some people, funding all manner of plastic surgery for the purpose of acquiring a svelte body is not a problem. If a wealthy patient is grossly overweight, yet has limited time for exercise – or, indeed, a limited inclination for it – they could resort to plastic surgery to do it for them in a passive way. Surgery would only make a partial difference, however. Following an exercise routine and observing proper nutritional standards will magnify the benefits of any cosmetic surgery.

Exercising engenders a positive cycle of feeling fit, and therefore being more active – and then eating better, and thus being more fit. When you are healthy, you eat healthily. When you are unhealthy, you eat poorly – things like convenience foods, often eaten largely for comfort. This again makes you more unhealthy still.

The minute you start working out and making yourself fitter and healthier, your whole cycle changes. You appetite decreases as you become more active, so it is a cumulative effect. This is probably one of the most important aspects of exercise. In addition, exercise releases endorphins, our body-grown narcotics, giving you a tremendous high. The best time to exercise is in the morning, before we go to work – but it takes willpower to get up an hour earlier.

In terms of what type of exercise, it really depends what one aims to achieve. If it is to build muscle, the exercise has to be strenuous. It doesn't need to be lengthy, but it does need to exceed your usual mental limit – if you do this you will push your physical limit higher. In other words you can always try harder than you think you can. Muscle-building exercise should be a stepped exercise: an initial warm up followed by repetitions using a combination of increasing weight and decreasing repetitions, with a last cycle at a weight one *below* the maximum – and for 12 repetitions. For instance, if you were doing a biceps exercise, you might take a 15 pound bar bell and do 12 repetitions, followed by a 17.5 pound bar bell for 10 repetitions, then a 20 pound bar bell for 8 repetitions, a 22.5 pound bar bell for 6 repetitions and, as a finale, the 20 pound bar bell for 12 repetitions.

Most of us can always push ourselves beyond what we think we can do and by doing this, we expand our ability to go to the next level. By doing so, we literally tear muscle cells and build new muscle.

When doing aerobic exercise, several cycles of intense activity are interspersed with slower cycles. For instance, if you were on a stationery treadmill, you would warm up for 2 minutes at 3.5 miles an hour, and then increase by 1 mile per hour every minute until you reach 7.5 miles per hour. Then you would go back to 4.5 miles per hour and repeat the cycle 4 times, only this time you would step up to 8.5 miles per hour – and so on until you feel that you have exceeded your mental capacity.

Each cycle should make you feel that you are using an effort level of 8 or 9 based on a scale of 1-10. The actual speed or weight is immaterial – everybody has their own scale and they know internally what level they are on. The very last cycle should see an effort level of 9 or 10.

Every effort is a mental as well as a physical phenomenon. This is the critical thing that many do not understand. We reach a point at which we think we are maximising our physical effort which is actually *below* our capability. If we drive ourselves beyond that point then we will stress muscle groups and create new muscle. If we stay within our comfort zone, our muscles accommodate and stay the same – no matter what the duration of exercise. The concept of having to do 30 or 40 minutes of aerobic exercise is baloney. You will get a better work out following the pattern above, which only takes about 21 minutes for the aerobics.

How necessary is this type of exercise? Only you can answer the question. Just remember that looking great requires effort. If, however, your ambitions are simply taking regular exercise in order to maintain your cardio-vascular health, then a less strenuous form of exertion can be adopted. Here are some of the main types:

Running & Jogging
By merely jogging, we can actually reduce the lean body mass. This is bad – one can age prematurely by literally cannibalising facial and upper body muscle to glucose. Jogging, therefore, can be counter-productive.

Running is probably one of the easiest exercises, but also one of the worst. The constant up-and-down motion loosens the facial and breast ligaments, and the loss of fat and muscle in the face and upper body gives a hollowed out and over-dieted look. Areas of fat resistant to diet and exercise are equally resistant to running. If you insist on pushing your cardio-vascular system, my advice is stick to the rowing machine.

People who insist on running should do so twice a week maximum, and alternate with other aerobic forms of exercise such as swimming or bicycling as well as muscle strengthening exercises. Aerobic exercise should be done 3 days a week and muscle strengthening 3 days a week.

Swimming

Swimming is good as it uses a lot of muscle – both upper body and lower body muscle. It puts minimal stress on the body because it is relatively weightless and, if you are a good swimmer, it is a great exercise.

At the gym

Personally I find gyms insanely boring. I also believe that people should have fun while they are exercising. My preferred option would be to do something that doesn't feel like exercise, such as kick boxing, jujitsu or yoga. That way, one would be engaging in strenuous exercise, all while learning a new skill and improving one's mental state. Martial arts are a beautiful synthesis of mental discipline and physical exercise.

In all disciplines, maintaining the same level of exercise is not beneficial. There are three rules of thumb to exercising properly:

Firstly, one should never do the same exercise every time because the body adapts to it, and adaptation prevents stimulus to the muscle and muscle growth. Secondly, one should alternate aerobic with muscle strengthening exercise on alternate days. By building muscle mass, one increases the metabolic rate. By increasing the metabolic rate we increase the rate at which we burn calories and therefore make it less likely that we will put on weight. Thirdly, always take one day off a week, and treat yourself to a diet and exercise vacation. Remember we don't get out of shape because of what we do on one day. It is what we do on the other six days that is the problem.

If you interested in learning how to exercise more effectively, read *Body for Life* by Bill Phillips, Harper Collins.

Diet

Why a section on diet? Well, you are what you eat — as well as what you smoke and drink. So if like T.S. Eliot you wake every morning to smoke a hearty breakfast, you will grow to look like him — or like Mick Jagger, Ozzy Osbourne, or any other celebrity you care to name who won't heed these obvious maxims.

For those who can't be a perfect 10 when it comes to living a healthy lifestyle, it doesn't hurt to know a thing or two about staying on the right side of the escalator – so that when you do feel in law-abiding mode you can reap the most benefit. The simple building blocks are in your diet (including nutritional supplements), water and exercise. The main things to avoid are smoking, alcohol (except a glass of wine with food) and sun. Everything we do should be designed to reduce the amount of anti-oxidants in our system. There are lots of good books on this (see *bibliography*), such as The Carbs Bible, The Zone, The South Beach Diet and The Perricone Prescription.

The main thing about diet is that people don't need to diet.
When a person starves themselves to lose weight, the body goes into a starvation mode and refuses to burn fat, saving it for a period of abstinence. It becomes like an animal in hibernation – it stores fat as a normal metabolic response. Starving the body of water also slows our basal metabolic rate and all these things make us gain weight. On the other hand if we don't eat properly we will eat ourselves. The right food and lifestyle helps to protect our body and make it work efficiently.

We are programmed to be foragers, so we should be constantly feeding ourselves. Six times a day would be the optimum – constantly eating, but not over-eating or eating the wrong foods. Eating on a regular basis keeps the metabolic pump functioning, cycling fat into glucose in the blood (provided that we are not eating excess calories). Portion size is critical. A portion of anything should be the size of your fist (e.g. a potato or an apple) or the size of your palm (e.g. a chicken breast or a fillet of fish). Remember that when you buy your food in a restaurant it is YOU, not the chef who decides how much you are going to eat. If you eat everything he puts on the plate, don't forget it was your choice.

The response of elevated blood glucose to food is delayed, so that a feeling of satiety often follows after we have eaten more calories than we require. Eating slowly or eating half of what is on the plate can help correct overeating. Other tricks to eating sensibly are to turn the bread basket away, drink water instead of sodas, and eating soups as your starter while you are waiting for the main course. Starchy foods like potatoes, bread and pastries contain high glycaemic carbohydrates and are easily converted into fat. To learn more about glycaemic indexes you should read *The Zone* by Barry Sears. (*see* bibliography)

Calories and Fast Food

Low-glycaemic carbohydrates are good. High-glycaemic carbohydrates rapidly convert into glucose in the blood stream, causing the insulin to rise and pushing the glucose into storage as fat, as well as preventing proper utilisation of body fat stores. In this scenario, one gets an insulin high followed by an insulin low which suggests the need to eat again. This in turn increases the appetite. So by eating high glycaemic carbohydrates we initiate a vicious cycle of insulin highs followed by lows that require further infusions of glucose. The ideal would be to have a constant level of insulin.

Low-glycaemic carbohydrates, such as green vegetables, will convert slowly into fructose – which will cause a gentle rise in insulin levels. Examples are Granny Smith Apples, avocadoes, broccoli, spinach and cauliflower, and all berries. Seldom-realised is that many fruits have concentrations of fructose which are rapidly converted into glucose, e.g. oranges, bananas and grapes. So concentrating on eating as much fruit and vegetables as you want is not necessarily a recipe for losing weight – although frankly it is much better than junk food which contains no fibre, no vitamins and often a lot of carcinogenic additives.

In addition many vegetables are rich in anti-oxidants which prevent cell damage. Examples are the oily products like olives, olive oil, coconut oil and fruits such as blueberries, strawberries, raspberries. Drinking green tea, herbal tea and decaffeinated tea or coffee has minimal effect on the insulin levels. Drinking regular coffee, on the other hand, will stimulate a burst of insulin.

In order for people to acquire more than a superficial understanding of low-glycaemic and high-glycaemic foods, I would recommend reading The South Beach Diet with its accompanying South Beach Recipe" book (see *Bibliography*).

The other food bible that I refer to is *Fast Food Nation*, which explains how fast food is manufactured and why it is bad. 'Fast Food' comprises nothing but unadulterated empty calories with no nutritional value. It is often high-fat, high-carbohydrate and low-fibre. I consider crisps and sodas such as cola to be as great a health risk as cigarettes. These are made by multi-billion pound corporations creating an artificial need where none exists. They also are the single most important cause of obesity in the Western World.

The English have a 'curse', if you will, of producing incredibly good-tasting items such as shortcakes, scones, clotted cream, jam and marmalade as well as various savoury pies, all of which are nutritionally unbalanced and I think explain a lot of the middle-age and old-age obesity in this country. Even though we are nowhere near as obese as the Americans, there is nothing worse for the figure than English afternoon tea, whether taken at Fortnum's or the Pierre next door to my New York Office at 800 Fifth Avenue. English High Tea is an absolutely glorious celebration of everything that is bad for the body – other than the drink tea itself. The tea alone would be very healthy, but everything else that goes with it is a complete and unmitigated disaster.

Many of our politicians seem to characteris e this middle aged spread: the likes of John Prescott, Gordon Brown, Michael Howard and so on. Tony Blair is in remarkably good shape and very youthful looking. American politicians tend to be fitter,

Republican or Democrat: Kerry and Bush are both typical.

What is needed is high street fast food that is nutritionally sound, low in calories, low-glycaemic and high-fibre. I think it is a great shame that one of the fastest-growing chains in the world is Starbucks, which mostly promotes coffee and pastries. Fortunately they serve tea also.

One caveat is that children and young adults should enjoy their food, excluding fast food. They can tolerate a much higher intake of carbohydrates. For example, I give my 14 year old son Sebastian (who is six foot three inches tall) as many milkshakes as he wants. He gets the calcium and the vitamin D which he needs for his bones. For children who don't like milk, give them ice-cream or chocolate milk instead. But this must be a treat and not a means to spoil them.

A sobering statistic is that there about 12 million candidates for weight loss surgery in the United States. They are now considering opening up paediatric surgical wards to cope with childhood obesity.

Health Supplements
This is not a book on health supplements and I am not a cardiologist or a nutritionist. I just read the books and listen to the advice, both good and bad, and this is my distillation of it. For

those who want a more exact guide please take a look at the bibliography.

However, remember that mono-unsaturated fatty acids, such as can be found in olive oil, are healthy, which is why the Greeks have such a low incidence of heart disease. Health supplements are essential, mainly because most of us may not remember to take all of our minerals and vitamins every day from our natural diet. All supplements are separated into vitamins and minerals which are catalysts for the body's metabolism. The former come in fat-soluble form (ADEK), which can be stored in the body, and in water-soluble form (which have to be replenished daily because they are excreted). Then there are minerals and finally food supplements such as anti-oxidants, as well as essential amino-acids and essential polysaccharides which counteract undesirable cell-damage. The rest are calorific building blocks such as essential fatty acids, protein and carbohydrate, which are used to build the tissue in our body and provide the energy to drive our metabolism. To keep our body toned we need to feed it with high quality protein throughout the day, since the body cannot store protein. Fibre is not metabolised but allows the bowels to contract efficiently and modulates the absorption of nutrients. Eating carbohydrate with protein and fibre slows its absorption.

For women, there are a number of especial must-haves such as calcium and iron. Women usually reach their highest level of bone calcium at the age of eighteen, after which it goes gradually down. In order to maintain a healthy level of calcium, women should consume milk and dairy products, and if they want or need to avoid these because of lactose intolerance or other allergies, they should take calcium supplement tablets. Because of the menstrual blood loss they need iron supplements to maintain their level of haemoglobin, which is the oxygen-carrying molecule of the blood and is primarily responsible for our exercise tolerance and energy level.

Before establishing a regime of supplement intake, however, it is worth noting that many of the products commonly sold on the market are simply flushed out of the system with zero benefit. This is because they are not formulated properly. Also, try to stick to organic products rather than processed foods, and eat ocean-caught fish rather than meat or farm fish as your primary protein source.

Vitamins should come in a bio-active form, produced from freeze-dried vegetables and then compacted into tablet form. In their synthetic form, vitamins have little nutritional value. Other essential supplement are anti-oxidants such as omega oils found in fatty fish, flax seed oil, olive oil and essential polysaccharides, such as aloe. Essential polysaccharides together with anti-oxidants protect us from affliction – colds, cancer, and actinic radiation from the sun. Antioxidants help to keep our skin young.

Nobody can succeed in dieting forever – everybody wants to have some chocolate cake occasionally. If you are forced on a diet that involves constant deprivation, you will inevitably fall off the wagon at some point and do what is natural to you – that is, enjoy your food. We are none of us designed to be anorexic – it's not a natural state of affairs nor is it remotely good for us, either from a health point of view or in the signals it gives to our body. One should choose one's diet so that it is always healthy and always good, yet we should never feel as if though we are actually on a diet.

If and when we do 'fall off the wagon', we shouldn't feel as if we are failures and degenerate back into slobs. Everybody falls off once in a while, and we must try to pick ourselves back up again and accept that fact that we are human. There is always the next day to be virtuous again, providing we actually mean it. I apply this philosophy to most things in life, including alcohol and the occasional cigar. I don't want be a healthy monk.

I am reminded of the wisdom of the Hispanic actor Antonio Banderas, who said once that the Spanish prize three things above all: good sex, good wine, and good sleep.

I am not sure what order he recommended taking these. Sex and sleep come naturally to us all. But wine, I feel, is an essential part of life: it helps with digestion, it's good for the heart and food tastes all the better for it.

THE **FUTURE**

The effect of plastic surgery on society

In the absence of conversation, we communicate with our face. The human face does broadcast a lot of messages. Sometimes, plastic surgery and Botox can restrict the natural ways we communicate these – and sometimes, the message is loud and clear: 'Yes I've had a facelift, yes I've had plastic surgery and no, I don't look anywhere near my age.'

People of a certain age who can't bear to have a wrinkle on their face often become the butt of jokes. But the alternative for them would be to look their age, which could spell the end of their career. It could also spell the end of them feeling good about themselves. Many people in the public eye go for the tight look. Even so, the skin relaxes after a while and the result is not so clearly visible. Yet many expect some longevity from their surgery: they are spending a lot of money and want the results to last. Barbara Walters, now seventy-three years old, wouldn't be able to carry on doing the job that she does if she looked her age and that goes for a lot of other people in broadcasting (it is said that TV ages a person by ten years – and makes them look ten pounds heavier too).

The fact is people who come to see the plastic surgeon are not interested in how he might alter their spontaneous facial expressions, rather they want him to address their concerns about a certain feature being too small or too large and in themselves sending out a wrong message – for example, a small chin suggests a passive personality or a down-turned mouth suggests a sour temperament. A large nose is not only unattractive, but may distract people from getting any message from your large eyes or beautiful smile, because they would be focused on the 'nose' rather than anything else. It is important to create harmony so that people focus on you, and your face as a whole, and not on one particularly jarring feature of your face. Remember the scene in *Austin Powers – The Spy Who Shagged Me* (1999) where Austin meets the Secret Agent with the Mole on his lip and can only keep exclaiming 'Mole'? Funny but completely true.

Facial expression is not what plastic surgery is about. You have to imagine that plastic surgeons look at a face as a static image. They are not looking at it with the notion of what happens when it moves, but rather as a piece of sculpture, rather like Michelangelo would look at proportions. The subtle interplay of facial muscle, connecting tissue and nerve that underpins the astonishing range of emotions and thoughts that we are broadcasting every waking moment is not part of the surgeon's remit. This is where we should fear to tread and is the reason why I keep away from the deep-plane, commando-style facelifts that are, in my opinion, more likely to produce the mask-like look. I do not do them because I cannot predict or control the expressive capacity of the face once it comes back together after surgery.

Plastic surgery junkies

There are people who, despite the pain and expense of plastic surgery become addicted to the lure of being able to tweak and refine their appearance. They are constantly looking for new ways to improve their face and body. Some of them look terrible – these are pathological addicts who are continually going under the knife. Mercifully, they are still a minority. As a plastic surgeon you run out of things you can offer them – providing you are observing your ethical duties to the patient. The surgeon certainly has a responsibility to those in thrall to narcissism to save them from drowning in the waters of the fountain. Such patients can usually continue with Botox and fillers, but after a while there is nothing more one can do for them.

If there is a significant risk that I can make someone look worse rather than better, then not only won't I operate on them but I also discourage them from seeking out some surgical cowboy who will.

The greatest danger with addiction to plastic surgery is that people end up with a facial disaster that is not merely uncorrectable but cannot be hidden from public display and ridicule either. Michael Jackson is a case in point. Such people are their own worst enemy and a living testimonial to the worst in plastic surgery.

There is a saying in surgery that the enemy of good is better.
A surgeon has to tread a fine line when operating on repeat patients. If someone comes in after they've had rhinoplasty and the result is fine with just a few minor imperfections, I would occasionally tell the patient that there is nothing I can do for them, because even though they could be made to look marginally better, it is not worth running the risk of making them look worse

This usually makes people realise they should leave it alone, but that is a hard thing for many to deal with. I have patients of my own who, even though they have a good result, will 'nitpick' it to death. Sometimes, I agree with them and go back and try to improve it. Other times I say this is the best I can do. Another response to this kind of nitpicking is to explain the natural asymmetry of the face.

When you get a facelift, it is akin to getting a new car – you notice every little scratch at first. It is the same effect with a new face – you scrutinise it for hours to see whether or not it's perfect. Suddenly you see that one eye is smaller than the other – what you don't realise is that one eye was *always* smaller than the other. This is why plastic surgeons always take 'before' and 'after' pictures of patients, so we can take them through the changes and help them understand these asymmetries. Often people don't realise that the two sides of their face are different. Generally, once patients 'wear' their new face in, they come to appreciate their asymmetries, but the operating table is definitely not the appropriate theatre for seeking perfection.

Another trap that people can fall into when engaging a plastic surgeon stems from the very English habit of wanting to keep the whole thing secret. Such patients will typically claim to be taking an extended holiday while actually booking into a clinic. The problem with this is that the element of subterfuge often detracts from the kind of consultation and research necessary for achieving the best results.

Mary Archer probably fell into the super-secretive trap. She had a very dramatic and clearly obvious facelift – with an excellent result – then returned determined to keep it a secret. When her sacked personal assistant revealed it, she sued her and, even more ridiculously, the judge ruled in her favour. Thankfully, the English climate of hypocrisy that clouds open discussion of plastic surgery is beginning to lift. This would be inconceivable in America where patients are more likely to give a party to show off their expensive new face to friends and, perhaps, a few enemies too. Although having cited the Americans as devoid of such hypocrisy, I have just seen Farah Fawcett on television claiming that in her entire life she has never undergone the stitch of a plastic surgeon.

Joan Collins, even though she spends most of her time abroad, is another woman afflicted with English hypocrisy. She maintains that she hasn't had any plastic surgery. If she hasn't, why make such a song and dance of it? There isn't any genetic, social, emotional or moral advantage in *not* undergoing plastic surgery. Those who can afford it but decline surgical enhancement are banking debauched currency when they try to make moral capital out of their choice. Such a choice has no more moral significance than a woman choosing not to perm her hair. Of course, those public figures who regularly visit their plastic surgeon, then publicly claim a la Farah Fawcett that they don't, are just as morally bankrupt. If such people have but don't want to talk about it, they should just tell inquiring or accusing journalists to mind their own business.

Is the beauty ideal synonymous with youth?

Not necessarily, is the short answer. There are some things youth gives you in beauty terms that you cannot get back, but many 20-25 year olds are going to look a lot more attractive when they are older. A freckly, gum-chewing girl with a pierced nose and a tattoo in the small of her back is no embodiment of beauty. Many gangly, badly-dressed teenagers become sophisticated, slimmed, toned adults. So there is a large window of time in which both men and women can improve with age as long as they consciously pursue that goal. A higher income and better clothes, grooming, hairstyle alone make the difference. Add some exercise and a good diet... Most young adults are on a budget and, although there are some 18-year-olds who know how to look sophisticated, they will have been brought up to cultivate this look and it is not natural to that age group.

The cult of youth is more pervasive today than ever before, which is one reason why people are much more intolerant of the signs of growing old than they were in the past. Our reference points then were also much narrower: people didn't travel and were not exposed to very much information on cosmetic surgery or, for that matter, to images that encouraged them to consider it. This is no longer the case. The genie is well and truly out of the bottle. We now know exactly how the select few, who secretly and seemingly magically used to defy the laws of nature, do it. Newspapers, magazines and websites freely discuss which celebrities have what bits nipped and tucked. There are now television programmes devoted to the subject, showing patients before, during and after their surgical enhancement.

So the long answer is much the same as the short answer. Older people are taking back from youth the beauty ideal that they hijacked in the 1950s and 60s. Surgical enhancement is one of the means by which they are doing it.

The impact of plastic surgery on society

Think not what plastic surgery did for society, but what society did for plastic surgery. Laurence Kirwan

Plastic surgery has become what it is today because of unprecedented public demand – it is assuredly not the case that plastic surgery moulded society in its own image. Doctors did not 'invent' plastic surgery: they devised solutions to problems people presented them. Just imagine if everybody was happy with ageing and nobody wanted to look any different, then the facelift would not exist as an operation. Plastic surgery itself doesn't suggest that we feel inadequate about how we look, it exists because we say 'I don't like the way I look, I want to look different'.

Mass media does do its best to popularise the issue, beaming it relentlessly through shows such as *Extreme Makeover* and *Hollywood Uncovered*, documentaries like *Dr. 9021* and dramas such as *Nip/Tuck*, so there is a kind of symbiosis here. Plastic Surgery is the 'monster' society created, and now in turn plastic surgery has influenced society through images in the media. But the primary demand has to come from the patient. Plastic surgeons don't advertise themselves and even where they do, people don't just stumble upon them. It is the desire of the patient that drives cosmetic surgery, pure and simple.

To illustrate this supply and demand, after the events of 9/11 some plastic surgeons didn't see any patients for 3 months – and some of them nearly went out of business. People had other priorities, other things on their mind, and didn't think of improving their looks. The plastic surgery industry in New York City ground to a halt as no one spent money on it.

When everybody came out of the shock, it had almost the reverse effect. Many people felt that if they were in danger of being victim to a terrorist attack even sitting at their desk, then they should make the most of their money and their time and indulge themselves. 'I might as well have a facelift now because I may not be here tomorrow' was the thinking. In times of cataclysms, be they natural or man-made, people stop thinking of plastic surgery – they even stop thinking of buying a new suit or car. But when society returns to normal, so does its demand for self-seeking indulgences.

Does plastic surgery affect the process of natural selection? Will enhanced people be attracted to other enhanced people – thus creating a plastic super race?

Well, not really, because as I have already noted surgery cannot affect one's genes. Nonetheless, there is a subtle effect in the way the cream of the crop are drawn to one another, and the surgically-enhanced are becoming harder to distinguish from the naturally young and beautiful. Thus, the cliché of older men dating younger women is becoming reversed as in the case of Demi Moore,

Melanie Griffith and Cameron Diaz to name a few. The men did it on money and power, whereas the woman are doing it on looks. Thus Mrs. Robinson of *Graduate* fame is alive and well, and looking just as good as Anne Bancroft did in the film.

We have examined how media shapes the perception of beauty but how does plastic surgery shape our perception of beauty? Men are so exposed to – one might say even *besieged* by a digitally enhanced image of beauty – that some find it hard to accept the imperfections of reality.

Women, on the other hand, are under constant pressure to conform to what they are told is a desirable way to look. The media, fashion and cosmetic conglomerate is a mega-industry with one purpose – to make money. This it does by constantly updating images of beauty, so that every year women (and men) flock back into to the shops to find new clothes, new make-up and perfume, new products and new fashions. To quote John Berger, 'the economic logic of fashion depends on making the old-fashioned look absurd'.

Fashion has penetrated everything, right down to the chair or sofa or beach-mat you are sitting on and there is nothing really that is around us that is not part of that complex. Even antiques and art of certain periods go in and out of fashion

Models have become role models. Such is the allure of the media-created celebrity that people actually go to plastic surgeons asking to be made to look like someone else. This is especially true for women, and the more attractive the woman, often the more insecure she tends to be.

As plastic surgery offers seemingly endless possibilities for enhancement, people are and will remain fascinated with its potential. Yet, in the midst of this potential for difference, what is occurring is a homogenisation of looks. The Asians want to look more Caucasian with occidental eyelids and stronger noses. The Africans want narrower noses, straighter hair and (in the case of Michael Jackson) lighter skin. The Caucasians want to be tanned, to have flatter, more Asian noses and upward tilts to their eyelids. Most Caucasian women want to be blonde. Everyone wants to be taller, me included. And everybody wants and needs liposuction.

There are some differences between the regions of the earth. Historically South American women have wanted smaller breasts and larger bottoms and Caucasians the opposite. However, the idea of having a more curvaceous bottom is now being appreciated in the Northern Hemisphere thanks to J-Lo and Kylie Minogue popularising the rear-end.

I think the culture of easy exposure has also made plastic surgery more imperative. Both sexes are exposing more flesh but especially women. On any high street the pants are getting so low that the butt-crack and the lower abdomen have become new erotic areas acceptable to put on public display. So far neither sex is yet flaunting their genitals – but such things are only a matter of time. Pornography is going mainstream; perversions normalised. You can see advertisements on the tube of fat middle-aged men being spanked by a dominatrix. The lingerie ads are all sexually explicit. There is now an entirely new field of cosmetic surgery called 'vaginal rejuvenation' to tighten the vagina and augment the G-spot, which supposedly rivals the clitoris as a trigger point for the female orgasm. Shaving of armpits and legs and bikini lines in women has led to the shaving of the whole body in men, and the classic bikini wax has shrunk to a landing strip or even nothing at all, leaving a 'go bare' attitude in both men and women.

The naked ape truly is becoming naked once again.

BIBLIOGRAPHY

The Naked Ape: A Zoologist's Study of the Human Animal, by Desmond Morris; Publisher: McGraw-Hill Companies, The (1967)

Fast Food Nation: The Dark Side of the All-American Meal by Eric Schlosser Publisher: Perennial; 1st edition (2002)

The Low-Carb Bible, Your All-In-One Guide to Successful Low-Carb Dieting, by Elizabeth M. Ward & Linda R. Yoakam, Publisher: Publications International, Ltd. (2003)

Patient Heal Thyself, by Jordan S. Rubin, Publisher: Freedom Press (2003)

Body for Life, by Bill Phillips and Michael D'Orso, Publisher: Harper Collins (1999)

The South Beach Diet, by Arthur Agatston M.D., Publisher: Rodale (2003)

The Perricone Prescription, by Nicholas Perricone, Publisher: Harper Collins (2002)

Aesthetic Plastic Surgery, by Thomas D. Rees, Publisher: W.B.Saunders (1980)

Plastic Surgery Chapter 1, Introduction to Plastic Surgery, by Joseph G. McCarthy, M.D. Publisher: W.B.Saunders (1990),

What Not To Wear, by Trinny Woodall & Susannah Constantine, Publisher: Weidenfield & Nicolson (2002)

Bernini by Wittkower, Publisher: Edizioni Electa (1998)

Other Books worth reading:
The Story of Art, by E.H. Gombrich; Publisher: Phaidon Press; 16th edition (1995)

The Nude: A Study in Ideal Form by Kenneth Clark Publisher: Doubleday; (January 1959)

Civilisation by Kenneth Clark, Publisher: Hermann; (1974)

Italian Renaissance Painting (Icon Editions) by James Beck, Publisher: Addison-Wesley Pub Co (1981)

The Fashion Book by Editors of Phaidon Press, Publisher: Phaidon Press; (1998)

Sylvain's Tahiti by Adolphe Sylvain, Publisher: Taschen; (2001)

A History of the Breast by Marilyn Yalom Publisher: Ballantine Books; (1998)

Body Watching by Desmond Morris Publisher: Jonathon Cape; (1985)

About Looking by John Berger. Publisher: Pantheon Books; (1980)

Scientific & Public Talks:
Laurence Kirwan, M.D., F.R.C.S., F.A.C.S.

The 'Executive Facelift', the 'Rejuvenation Rhinoplasty' and the treatment of 'Varicose Veins & Spider Veins' and 'Hair Loss & Hair Restoration in Women' at the Body Beautiful Show at the Café Royal, London, September 25 and 26, 2004.

'New Soft Tissue Fillers' at the 'Hot Topics Section' of the Annual meeting of the American Society of Plastic Surgeons 10/09/04 – 10/13/04 PLASTIC SURGERY 2004. Pennsylvania Convention Center, Philadelphia, PA

The American Society for Aesthetic Plastic Surgery 04/28/05 – 05/04/05 ASAPS/ASERF. Annual Meeting: Ernest N. Morial, Convention Center, New Orleans, LA.

General Publications:

Hair Transplantation in Women: The New Frontier, by Laurence Kirwan MD. May/ June 2004. Aesthetic Trends & Technologies trade journal for physicians

Anchor Thighplasty, Aesthetic Surgery Journal, 24/1 pp 61-64, January/February 2004.

Anchor Thigh-plasty ANZ J Surg. 2003:73, (Suppl) p.226. Presented at the 13th International Congress, International Confederation for Plastic, Reconstructive and Aesthetic Surgery, Sydney, Australia. Aug. 14, 2003.

My Mole Book: A children's information book by Laurence Kirwan with illustrations by Richard Cole, 2003. My Mole Book.

Addressing Acne, Plastic Surgery Products Magazine by Laurence Kirwan, MD, FRCS, FACS, March, 2003. View article.

Three-Dimensional Liposculpture of the Iliac Crest and Lateral Thigh Aesthetic Surgery Journal, 17, 334-336, September / October 1997

Breast Surgery Publications:

Breast Augmentation in the Ptotic Breast, Aesthetic Trends Magazine, September/October 2003.

Lollipop Mastopexy, ANZ J Surg. 2003:73, (Suppl) p.224. Presented at the 13th International Congress, International Confederation for Plastic, Reconstructive and Aesthetic Surgery, Sydney, Aug. 14, 2003

A Classification and Algorithm for Treatment of Breast Ptosis: Aesthetic Surgery Journal, 22:355-363, July/August 2002.

Inverted Nipple and Nipple Reconstruction: The 'Parachute' Flap: Canadian Journal of Plastic Surgery, 7(5):233-236, September/October 1999

Simultaneous Areolar Mastopexy/
Breast Augmentation – The SAMBA™
Procedure, Surgical Strategies For The
Ptotic Breast: Aesthetic Surgery
Journal, 19, 34-39, January/February
1999

Brief Communication: Two Cases Of
Apparent Silicone Allergy: Plast
Reconst Surg, 96:236, 1995

Expert Panels, Symposia, Lectures
Recent Expert Panels:

IPRAS World Congress, 2003 Sydney,
Australia: Thursday August 14th.
Expert Panel: Mastopexy with
Augmentation Mammaplasty. Chair:
Tom Biggs. With Joao Sampaio Goes,
Gusztav Gulyas, Laurence Kirwan.
Aesthetic Course 59. Laurence Kirwan:
Simultaneous Areolar Mastopexy/
Breast Augmentation – The 'SAMBA'
Procedure.

Expert Panel: 'Augmentation
Mastopexy - Controlling Scar
Perceptibility and Nipple Shape.' May
2nd, 2002

Symposia:

IPRAS World Congress, 2003 Sydney,
Australia: Course Presentation:
'Management of Breast
Ptosis/Augmentation of the Ptotic
Breast. Presented at the 13th
International Congress, International
Confederation for Plastic,
Reconstructive and Aesthetic Surgery,
August 14th, Sydney,Australia.

Fourth Annual Symposium:
'Management of Breast
Ptosis/Augmentation of the Ptotic
Breast, The Aesthetic Meeting 2004
Annual Meeting of ASAPS and
ASERF, Vancouver Convention Center,

April 15-21, Vancouver, Columbia.

Third Annual Symposium:
'Management of Breast Ptosis
/Augmentation of the Ptotic Breast,
'Annual Meeting of the American
Society for Aesthetic Plastic Surgery,
John P. Hynes Veterans Memorial
Convention Center Boston, MA., May
15-21, 2003.

Second Annual Symposium:
'Management of Breast
Ptosis/Augmentation of the Ptotic
Breast,' Annual Meeting of the
American Society for Aesthetic Plastic
Surgery, Caesars Palace, Las Vegas,
Nevada. April 30th, 2002

First Annual Symposium: Simultaneous
Areolar Mastopexy/Breast
Augmentation – The SAMBA
Procedure, Surgical Strategies For The
Ptotic Breast: Aesthetic Meeting 2000,
Scientific Meeting of The American
Society for Aesthetic Plastic Surgery,
Hilton Towers, New York, New York,.
May 2001

4th Annual Symposium on
Simultaneous Areolar Mastopexy /
Breast Augmentation: Dr Kirwan
presented on the SAMBA Procedure:
Surgical Strategies For The Ptotic
Breast, at the 70th Annual Scientific
Meeting of The American Society of
Plastic Surgeons, Orlando, Florida,
United States, November 5th, 2001.

Third Annual Symposium:
Simultaneous Areolar
Mastopexy/Breast Augmentation – The
SAMBA™ Procedure, Surgical
Strategies For The Ptotic Breast:69th
Annual Scientific Meeting of The
American Society of Plastic Surgeons,
Los Angeles. October 2000

Second Annual Symposium:

Simultaneous Areolar Mastopexy/Breast Augmentation – The SAMBA™ Procedure, Surgical Strategies For The Ptotic Breast: 68th Annual Scientific Meeting of The American Society of Plastic Surgeons, New Orleans. October 1999

First Annual Symposium: Simultaneous Areolar Mastopexy/Breast Augmentation - The SAMBA™ Procedure, Surgical Strategies For The Ptotic Breast: 67th Annual Scientific Meeting of The American Society of Plastic Surgeons, Boston. October 1998

Simultaneous Areolar Mastopexy/Breast Augmentation – The SAMBA™ Procedure, Surgical Strategies For The Ptotic Breast: The 2nd Congress Of The European Academy Of Cosmetic Surgery, London. May 9th, 1998.

Lectures

Aug. 14, 2003, Kirwan, L., Lollipop Mastopexy, ANZ J Surg. 2003:73, (Suppl) p.224. Presented at the 13th International Congress, International Confederation for Plastic, Reconstructive and Aesthetic Surgery, Sydney.

An Algorithm for Augmentation of the Ptotic Breast: Breast Surgery and Body Contouring Symposium, Eldorado Hotel, Santa Fe, NM. Sponsor:

Plastic Surgery Educational Foundation and American Society for Aesthetic Plastic Surgery. August 23rd and 24th 2001.

Wise-pattern Areolar Mastopexy Breast Augmentation: The 'WAMBA' procedure: Breast Surgery and Body Contouring Symposium, Eldorado Hotel, Santa Fe, NM. Sponsor: Plastic Surgery Educational Foundation and American Society for Aesthetic Plastic Surgery. August 23rd and 24th 2001.

Dr Kirwan's web sites:
www.drkirwan.com for facial plastic surgery and body contouring and hair restoration
www.surgicalbreastenhancement.com for cosmetic breast surgery
www.dermiscenter.com for non-surgical services
www.kirwanveincenter.com for injection therapy of varicose veins and spider veins

Contact Information

In the USA:
605 West Avenue
Norwalk, CT
USA 06850
Ph: (203) 838-8844
Fax:(203) 853-1862
Email Dr. Kirwan
fcps.lk@att.net
Also in the USA at:
800 Fifth Avenue, Suite 202
(corner of 61st St.)
New York, NY 10021
Ph: (212) 838 8844
Fax:(203) 853-1862
Email Dr. Kirwan
In the UK:
112 Harley Street
London W1G 7JQ
Ph: (020) 7935 8844
(after 2:00 p.m.)
Fax: (020) 7908 3879
Email Dr. Kirwan
fcps.lk@att.net

Dr Kirway does not perform consultations by email. Please contact his office for an apointment.

ARTNIK '04/5

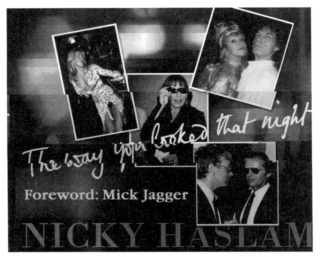

The Way You Looked That Night
Nicky Haslam

Nicky Haslam is virtually the in-house designer for high society. His work combined with a chameleon-like ability to mix as easily with rock stars as royalty has given him a Polaroid-eye for capturing the reality beneath the pose of celebrity. In *The Way You Looked That Night*, he opens up his private photo albums to share his record of 30 years of high living around the world.

Nicky Haslam's credo for design is "to make people look more beautiful and feel happier". His book has exactly that effect on the reader.

Mick Jagger writes a witty, insightful foreword.

PRICE	£20
PUB DATE	Feb 14 2005
BIND	Hardback
SIZE	314mm x 258 mm
EXTENT	98pp
	countless colour + B/W photos
ISBN	1-903906-40-7

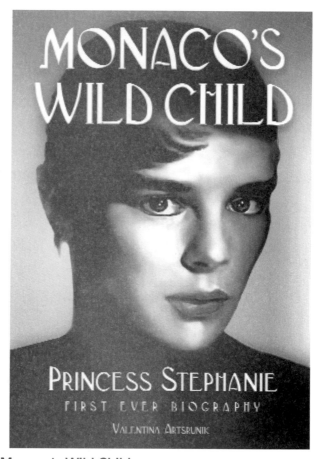

Monaco's Wild Child
Valentina Artsrunik

Monaco's Wild Child is the first ever biography of Stephanie of Monaco – a royal hellraiser who rivals Catherine the Great. She was dubbed by *The Sun* as "the trailer-trash princess". Certainly a woman who went from the fast lane into the farce one.

Valentina Artsrunik charts Stephanie's tumultuous life from riches to designer rags, taking in the men, the drink, the drugs, the rehab clinics... The author – who has lived in Monte Carlo – does not sensationalise but paints a human portrait of this complex, turbulent, fiercely independent woman.

TITLE	Monaco's Wild Child
AUTHOR	Valentina Artsrunik
PRICE	£14.99
PUB DATE	Oct 29 2004
BIND	Hardback
SIZE	198mm x 129 mm
EXTENT	256pp
	16pp insert colour + B/W photos
ISBN	1-903906-34-2

If a picture is worth a thousand words, a book is worth a thousand pictures

PUBLISHER
Artnik
341b Queenstown Rd, SW8 4LH
+44 (0) 20 7498 1257
artnikbooks@dsl.pipex.com
www.artnik.org

DISTRIBUTION & SALES
Airlift
Enfield, EN3 7NL UK
+(44) 020 8804 0400
orders@airlift.co.uk
www.airlift.co.uk